Meditation for Beginners

A Practical Guide to Start Meditating

Quiet Your Mind, Reduce Stress and Anxiety, Sleep Better, and Improve Focus with Proven and Time-Tested Guided Meditations

Mind, Body, and Spirit Masterclass

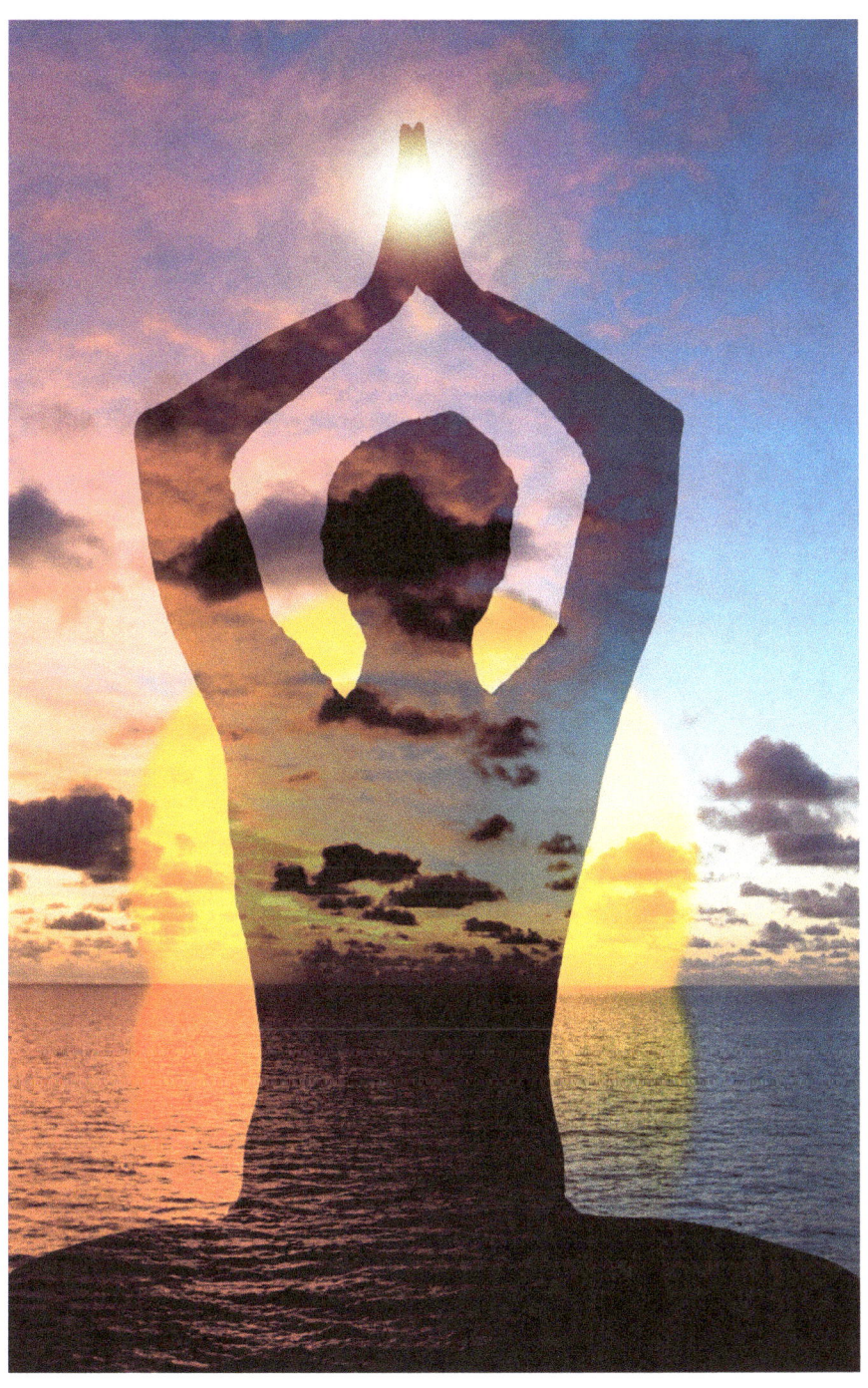

© Copyright 2022 - Mind, Body, and Spirit Masterclass -All rights reserved.

The following Book is reproduced below with the goal of providing information that is as accurate and reliable as possible. Regardless, purchasing this Book can be seen as consent to the fact that both the publisher and the author of this book are in no way experts on the topics discussed within and that any recommendations or suggestions that are made herein are for entertainment purposes only. Professionals should be consulted as needed prior to undertaking any of the action endorsed herein.

This declaration is deemed fair and valid by both the American Bar Association and the Committee of Publishers Association and is legally binding throughout the United States.

Furthermore, the transmission, duplication, or reproduction of any of the following work including specific information will be considered an illegal act irrespective of if it is done electronically or in print. This extends to creating a secondary or tertiary copy of the work or a recorded copy and is only allowed with the express written consent from the Publisher. All additional right reserved.

The information in the following pages is broadly considered a truthful and accurate account of facts and as such, any inattention, use, or misuse of the information in question by the reader will render any resulting actions solely under their purview. There are no scenarios in which the publisher or the original author of this work can be in any fashion deemed liable for any hardship or damages that may befall them after undertaking information described herein.

Additionally, the information in the following pages is intended only for informational purposes and should thus be thought of as universal. As befitting its nature, it is presented without assurance regarding its prolonged validity or interim quality. Trademarks that are mentioned are done without written consent and can in no way be considered an endorsement from the trademark holder.

Table of Content

Introduction 11

Meditation: What It is and What It Isn't 15

The Main Meditation Techniques 21

Traditional Meditation 22

Intentional Meditation 23

Transcendental Meditation 23

Mindfulness Meditation 24

Walking Meditation 25

Kundalini Meditation 26

Dynamic Meditation 26

Active and Passive Meditation 29

How to Start Meditating 35

Meditation and Routine 45

Where to Meditate and How Long 49

At Home 50

Outdoors 51

Meditation Schools or Specialized Centers 52

Special Locations 54

Breathing and Meditation 59

Ujjayi breathing 62

Kapalabhati Breathing 64

Relaxation Breathing 66

Diaphragmatic Breathing 68

Calming Breathing 70

Breathing for Positivity 71

Alternate Nostril Breathing 75

What Do You Need to Meditate? 79

The 9 Benefits of Meditation 87

Tips for Getting Started with Meditation 95

The 11 Tips for Meditating Better 101

The 13 Most Common Mistakes 109

Step-By-Step Meditations 121

Short Meditation - 1 Minute 122

Short Meditation - 3 Minutes 125

Short Meditation - 5 Minutes 127

Short Meditation for Gratitude - 5 Minutes 129

Short Morning Meditation - 3 Minutes 132

Meditation for Better Sleep - Short - 5 Minutes 134

Meditation to Reduce Anxiety - Short - 5 Minutes 136

Meditation to Reduce Stress - 10 Minutes 139

Mind-Body Connection Meditation - 5 Minutes 142

Meditation to Calm Your Mind - 10 Minutes 144

Conclusion 149

Introduction

Hello and welcome,

I am very happy that you have chosen my book to begin your journey to the discovery of the wonderful world of meditation. My name is Anja and I do coaching and counseling for those who need to rebalance their body, mind, and spirit. I cover topics such as Chakras, Meditation, Yoga, Crystal Therapy, and much more. In addition to my various books, you can find insights on these closely related topics on my Youtube channel, where you can ask me your questions for answers. This is the link to the channel which is called "Mind, Body & Spirit."

https://www.youtube.com/channel/UC5DxslTyhtdH5iQo1UtkO9Q

Now you know a little more about myself, let's get back to meditation. If you have decided to buy this book, you have most likely heard about meditation from many different sources around you, you would probably like to get the fantastic benefits everyone is describing, but you have no idea how to get started. It sounds complicated to you, something that is not in your chords, and that you don't fully understand. Don't worry! You are in the right place.

In this book, you will find everything you need to know to start meditating on your own at home and start enjoying the enormous benefits of meditation in a relatively short time. This is a manual entirely designed for beginners, so you will find detailed information for starting from scratch with the practice. Everything will be explained thoroughly so that it will be understood effortlessly even by those with really zero experience, and it will also be full of tips and suggestions that are always extremely useful when approaching something new for the first time.

You will find some theory in the book, just to do the necessary background such as, for example, understanding what meditation is, what it is really for, and what kinds of benefits it can bring to your life. Otherwise, the information you will find will be practical. In fact, I will explain many things that you will not just read about but will have to apply. I am referring to explanations on how to create your own meditation space, rather than how to breathe, and even complete step-by-step scripts on how to do your first meditations.

As in all other areas of life, it is acting that makes the difference. Action causes a reaction. So, it will not be enough for you to just read the book, if you want the benefits you will have to put the various steps and suggestions into practice. Not only that! You will have to persevere daily and treat meditation as a muscle to be trained. A daily workout, even if only a few minutes long, will bring you incredible results even in a quite short space of time.

Well, I would say that with the premises we are done, so we can set off on our journey to discover the wonderful world of meditation and all its benefits. You are about to discover and experience for yourself why there are so many people talking about this tool that is incredible for well-being, serenity, and happiness.

EVERYONE CAN MEDITATE!

EVERYONE SHOULD MEDITATE!

Meditation: What It is and What It Isn't

The term meditate comes from the ancient Latin word "meditari" which means to think, reflect and study.

By the term meditate, in a broad sense, we mean "to quiet the mind". Meditation is a state of deep peace in which the mind quiets down while still remaining alert.

The main goal of meditation is to bring all our attention right to ourselves to achieve deep inner peace and gain great self-awareness.

Meditation is a very powerful tool, but at the same time, it is very simple to use. To master it in the best way all it takes is perseverance in practicing it, just as I mentioned in the introduction. It will be through practice that you will be able to see the first results. Don't be frightened by this idea of constant practice. You might think that it will take up time you don't have or that you won't be able to integrate it into your daily routine. This is not the case at all.

The daily practice might take up as little as 5 minutes a day, but it would bring huge changes to your life in such a gentle way that it would become part of your routine without you almost noticing it.

Meditating makes us feel good about ourselves, and feeling good about ourselves is a condition that everyone should aspire to, in my opinion. That is why I believe that meditation is a practice suitable for everyone and not reserved for a select few. I also consider it an easy practice because I believe that anyone, with a little practice, can achieve the state of peace and self-awareness required to meditate, regardless of age or life experiences.

The benefits you can achieve by consistently practicing meditation are really many and incredible. It reduces stress levels, brings peace and harmony to the body and mind, strengthens mental and physical health, provides relief from chronic physical pain, improves sleep quality, gives serenity, helps you achieve greater awareness of your body and mind, and also awareness of who we are in our wholeness deep inside ourselves.

Meditation is a doorway to our roots, helping us to root ourselves, anchor ourselves, be present in the "here and now" and be centered.

This does not mean sitting for hours in a certain position, like that of the statue or that of the Buddha. In fact, you might find yourself meditating while doing something else. Maybe you are walking and without even realizing it you might be in a meditative state. It might happen to you when you are in contact with a natural element that you are particularly comfortable with. For example, immerse in the water, while bathing or swimming, you might be in a meditative state. In fact, let's say that the term doing meditation is a bit of a stretch; it would be more correct to say being in meditation, being in a meditative state.

A great many scientific studies have shown how much the mind changes after meditation. During meditation, our brain stops processing information and becomes quiet. Therefore, meditation leads to a deep state of physical and mental stillness. During meditation, the mind is calm and quiet but still alert.

This thoughtless state of peace and awareness cannot come if you concentrate on not thinking. During your first attempts at meditation, you tend to repeat to yourself, "I must not think, I must not think, I must not think!" Tough, you end up having the opposite effect and feeling worse than when you started. This is normal the first few times. That is why it is important not to give up, you have to keep trying and practicing. The state of mindless awareness will come slowly. With constant practice, you will create this state of inner peace, where you stay in touch with the pure essence of what you are in the present moment.

By "what you are in the present moment," I do not mean whether you are male or female, whether your name is Sarah or John, whether you are 20 or 60, whether you are happy, sad, angry, or tired. I am really referring to simply being in that moment, existing, breathing, a simple "I Am," "I Am Here." You are simply a presence in your body. This is meditation.

Meditation is like a muscle and it has to be trained, remember that for every action there is always a reaction, so if you meditate you will always enjoy the benefits. You just need to start with a few minutes a day. One minute, then two, then three, then five... maybe the results won't come right away, but slowly the repetition will change your unconscious mind and that will help you a lot. It will improve your quality of life immensely.

By now you should have understood what meditation is, but, for the avoidance of doubt, let's also see what it is not. All the talk about meditation has ended up distorting many people's ideas, so let's clarify them a bit.

Meditation is not a religious practice, but a practice to get in touch with one's spirituality. Religion and spirituality are two very different things. You are a spiritual being living in a physical body, often the hectic life makes you lose sight of your spirituality, and with meditation you go and get back in touch with it, it puts you back in touch with your spirit, with your spiritual part. Religion, on the other hand, is what binds a person to what they consider divine or sacred. Meditation is indeed used as a practice by many religions, but it is not in itself a religious practice.

Meditation is not a tool to achieve supreme enlightenment. Buddha's story is certainly fascinating and perhaps, with time and a lot of practice, you can achieve deep enlightenment, but there is no guarantee. That is not why you should practice meditation, you should practice it because it makes you feel good. If you set out in search of enlightenment, and you don't see tangible results in that area in a short time, you will give up, depriving yourself of a huge opportunity to live a better life.

In the next few chapters, we will dive into most of the concepts that I have merely mentioned in this first chapter to give you an understanding of what meditation is and how it can change your life for the better.

The Main Meditation Techniques

Many different meditation techniques have developed throughout history in different geographical areas, following different philosophies and traditions. They all are techniques with quite different applications. The advantage is that with so many different techniques, everyone can find the method that suits him best.

In my opinion, all this abundance of techniques ends up creating so much confusion in the heads of beginners, to the point of scaring them off and keeping them away from meditation. So, I would like to provide you with some explanations to easily and quickly clear any confusion you might have.

There are 3 techniques that I think are fundamental and I consider them the main ones for a beginner to start with. The choice of one of the 3 depends on the goal the beginner wants to achieve but also on what is closest to his personality and his way of being. I am referring to traditional meditation, intentional meditation, and transcendental meditation.

I will briefly describe all three so that you can have a clear idea about the main characteristics of each one. At the end of the chapter, I will also mention the other major techniques so that you will be familiar with them, but I recommend further study only when you have become a little more experienced in the practice.

Traditional Meditation

It is also called classical meditation or Zen meditation. To be clear, it is the classic seated meditation, usually cross-legged, that everyone thinks of when meditation is mentioned. The basis of this meditation is breath and stillness. You sit and watch your thoughts go by whilst listening to your breathing. Your mind is focused on the present moment.

The main benefits you get from this meditation technique are:

- Greater self-control

- Excellent observation skills

- Deep self-awareness

This technique helps you eliminate:

- Fear

- Insecurity

Intentional Meditation

Intentional meditation is also called aware meditation or "Vipassana." This term comes from ancient Indian and means "vision" or "looking deeply into things."

It is called intentional because it is based on awareness of our breathing. You practice it by focusing all your attention on an object and its movements. The object can be material or immaterial, that is, it can also be a vision, a visualization.

You focus on a specific image and you do it by nurturing a state of mind. It is intentional and conscious, you practice it to attract a certain result. You focus on a mental demand and a state of mind. The affirmation of what you want is your intention. Your intention is what you have to repeat in your meditation.

The main benefit of this technique is the elevation of your spirituality to a higher level, and from that higher level you can enjoy a new view of life, you gain a much more enlightened view of things.

Transcendental Meditation

Transcendental meditation is practiced by repeating a Mantra, that is, a special phrase or word to be repeated several times during the practice. First of all, it is important to find the Mantra that suits you best, and then it is necessary to recite it with your eyes closed for a certain time during the day. This mantra keeps the mind busy allowing the being to calm down, relax, and achieve inner peace.

The main benefits one gets from this meditation technique are:

- Harmony with our innermost self

- Inner peace

- Tranquility

- Harmony with the world around us

There are, as I mentioned at the beginning of the chapter, so many other meditation techniques. Aside from the three main ones that I recommend you focus on, for the time being, there are four others that, in my opinion, are worth mentioning for your knowledge and, perhaps, for future study when you will become a little more confident with meditation. They are mindfulness meditation, walking meditation, kundalini meditation, and dynamic meditation.

Mindfulness Meditation

This meditation technique is a Western-style revision of intentional meditation. Its practice is based on 3 cornerstones:

1. Focus on the present: here and now

2. Observe without judging

3. Analyze your emotions transparently, without preconceptions

The main benefit of this technique is total acceptance of yourself accompanied by deep self-awareness, which together allows you to free yourself from pain.

The basis of this practice is to be guided by feelings and emotions instead of thoughts. It is considered particularly suitable for those with the need to manage states of anxiety.

Walking Meditation

This practice is performed precisely by walking and its creation is attributed to Buddha himself during his awakening as he walked barefoot across India. As you physically move your body from one place to another by walking, meditation allows you to empty your mind of superfluous thoughts. You arrive, therefore, at your destination with a clearer and more organized mind than when you left.

The main benefits you gain from this meditation technique are:

- Finding peace daily through movement

- Organizing thoughts

- Disciplining the mind

Kundalini Meditation

This meditation technique is a bit more complicated than the others because it takes place in multiple sessions. Each session should awaken the energy of one Chakra and accentuate its benefits. There are seven main Chakras, so we are talking about at least seven sessions. If you are interested in learning more about Chakras, I have written a book about it, easily available in the main online bookstores.

Going back to meditation, kundalini energy is an energy that is spirally twisted at the base of the spine and is released by activating the Chakras.

The benefit of awakening this energy is an immense, very deep joy that flows from the center of your being as a result of full self-realization.

Dynamic Meditation

This technique is part of those techniques called active meditation, just like walking meditation. Its practice requires movement and expression. It is practiced by freeing your deepest emotions and expressing them through the movements of your body. It is possible to do this, for example, through dance (even frenetic dance) using each movement to channel the feelings and emotions that pervade you. As a result of this expression, you can better appreciate silence and calm.

Active and Passive Meditation

In the previous chapter, I covered what you can consider the main meditation techniques. There is another distinction to be made in the area of meditation that I think is very useful to know, even as a beginner, to have a totally clear idea about the various aspects of what it really means to meditate. I am referring to active and passive meditation. I find it important to clarify this point because there is always so much confusion and so many misconceptions about the concept of meditation. Let's see what the difference is and which one is the best option between the two.

We talked in the previous chapter about walking meditation but there are a lot of other examples of active meditation. The first example that comes to my mind is Yoga because I practice it regularly, but for many people, it is the sport they most like to practice that brings them into a meditative state. For some it is running, it is brisk walking by the sea, it is surfing or canoeing or perhaps hiking surrounded by nature.

When you play a sport you love, you enter a flow that generates gamma-type brain waves, which are the waves the brain emits during the meditative state. Very often the sports you love are practiced in contact with nature, and this creates a deep state of contemplation that really puts you in a state very similar to traditional meditation. The state described is only similar tough because traditional meditation is passive. In both cases you are in the flow, you emit gamma waves, you are present in the "here and now", and you are connected to what you are doing. Although these two states have so many similarities, they are actually profoundly different.

Body and mind are deeply linked and connected. So, if the body is doing something like hiking, running, or surfing, that is, it is moving, the mind follows and moves too. When you move your senses are turned outward to pick up the world around it in which you are moving and your mind is in motion to process all the information coming from your senses. In passive meditation, your senses are turned inward to look inside yourself, it is on your inner part that the focus goes.

Having your senses turned outward makes you a victim of the thousands of distractions of the world around you and this prevents you from entering a meditative state in the true sense of the word, that is, a deep meditative state.

The only way you can slow down the mind and reach the deep meditative state is to stop the body from moving. In passive meditation you are still and so the mind can slow down but in active meditation, with the body moving the mind follows, moving in turn.

So, active meditation can definitely work, but it cannot be your only form of meditation if you want to get the typical results of passive meditation. It is certainly better than not meditating completely, but you cannot expect the results that even a few minutes a day of passive meditation can give you.

Active meditation has no precise technique, unlike the various passive forms that have precise techniques on how to sit, how to breathe, eyes closed, attention turned inward, and so on. This is because it is not a true form of meditation, but only a pleasurable state that resembles meditation.

In passive meditation, the senses are turned inward and a state of stillness for the body and mind must be sought. A state of concentration, awareness, and presence in the "here and now." It is the attainment of this state that allows you to enjoy the benefits of meditation, and only passive meditation allows you to reach this state. You reach a totally different state of consciousness and awareness than the one you can achieve with active meditation, which is why the results of the two techniques are not comparable and are very far apart.

Passive meditation allows you to reach a state of pure mindless awareness, a state in which you are alert but deeply relaxed. In this state you are centered, grounded, and rooted. You are in a state of deep relaxation, peace, and harmony that only passive meditation can give you. You cannot reach this state with active meditation because your attention is focused on an outside world full of distractions.

So, I would say that if you have to choose only one form of meditation the best one is passive meditation, where you sit in silence, still, looking inward. Choosing passive meditation is the main point, then you can repeat a mantra to yourself, focus on the breath, an image, or an emotion, whatever form of passive meditation suits you best. It doesn't matter which passive meditation technique you use, the important thing is to achieve a different state of consciousness than usual, a relaxed state of mindless awareness, a state of peace of mind and harmony. Only by reaching the state that passive meditation can give you, you will be able to enjoy the benefits of meditation in your daily life.

If you feel like adding some active meditation to this, it can only do you good, but active meditation alone is not enough to help you achieve the state of well-being that passive meditation can give you.

Do you remember how I concluded the introduction to this book? Everyone can meditate, but most importantly ...
EVERYONE SHOULD MEDITATE!

How to Start Meditating

Personally, I have been practicing meditation daily for many years, so most of the tips and advice you will find on these pages have been tested by my own direct experience.

I said before that meditation is a state of concentration, deep listening to self, and presence in the "here and now", whilst being vigilant at the same time. When meditating, we are focused on something, but at the same time, we are relaxed. You might go so far as to say that we are in a "passive" state. As we analyzed in the previous chapter, there are 2 stages of meditation, active and passive, and they are very different from each other. When we feel we are meditating while walking, running, or cooking, we are in a state of active meditation, a meditation in which distractions are involved. In passive meditation, we are sitting, our eyes closed, and focusing exclusively on one thing, turning our senses inward, and not on the outside world as in active meditation. From the detailed description of the dedicated chapter and the brief summary I have given you in the previous lines, you should have understood that you are here to learn passive meditation, the active one will then come on its own according to your time and habits if you wish.

As I mentioned to you earlier, everyone can meditate and everyone who meditates gets enormous benefits. So, don't be discouraged, don't be afraid you won't succeed and don't listen to the skeptics who repeat, "Are you sure you want to do it? No, no! Meditation is not for me!"

So, how do you start meditating?

1. Posture

One of the fundamental aspects of meditation is the way of sitting or meditation posture. I feel like saying that often for those who are just starting out and are absolute beginners, a "perfect" posture is not so fundamental, but there are unavoidable elements of posture that it is best to respect from the beginning.

You must be seated, not necessarily with crossed legs. Your spine needs to be straight, but not rigid.

If you decide to start meditating sitting on the floor with your legs crossed, it is very useful to have a meditation cushion to put under your buttocks so that it supports your back and avoids straining it. You can also use a regular pillow to start with. Over time you will probably prefer to use a meditation pillow (there are many and you will have to choose the one that best suits your needs) for comfort in maintaining your posture. The purpose of the pillow is to make sure that your hips are positioned higher than your knees and that the position is comfortable without straining your back or tiring yourself out. The first few times, you will most likely feel tired anyway, but with time, repetition, and training this will no longer be the case.

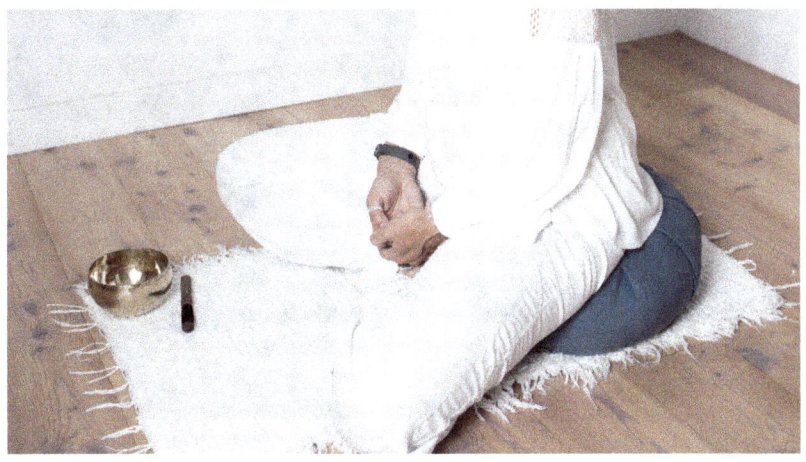

You may also decide to start meditating while sitting on a chair instead of on the floor. In this case, you should sit leaning against the backrest, with your back straight but not stiff, your legs not crossed, and your feet firmly on the ground (rooted). If the backrest does not make you comfortable or does not allow you to sit upright, then do not lean back, sit with your back straight, not stiff, and your legs not crossed, with your feet firmly rooted on the ground.

If, on the other hand, you decide to start meditating sitting on the floor, but on your knees, choose a cushion of those on which you can sit astride so that you still maintain a comfortable position that does not strain your back.

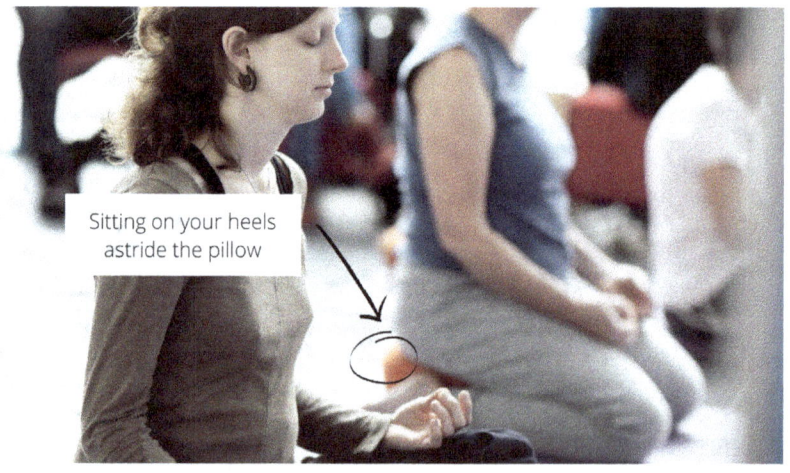

Sitting on your heels astride the pillow

Your hands, in whatever position you choose to sit, rest on your thighs or knees with palms up or down, as you are most comfortable.

2. Close Your Eyes

Close your eyes and take a moment to really begin to immerse yourself in the practice. This is your preparation for meditation. Eliminating visual stimuli will make it easier for you to begin this immersion inside yourself. So, close your eyes and …

3. Focus

Start focusing on something. There are so many things you can focus on. To get started, I recommend focusing on the most common and simplest one. Starting in the simplest way possible is always the best choice for mastering something new. When you have gained the necessary experience, you can move on to focus on whatever you prefer.

The most common and simple thing to start focusing on is the breath. You have to start by focusing on the flow of your breath, without trying to alter it. You have to let it flow and just observe its flow. You have to concentrate on the breath by observing its flow, visualizing it, and feeling it.

During meditation, some people are better at observing, some people are better at visualizing, some people are better at concentrating on the feelings that arise at the physical level, and some people are better at concentrating on the feelings that arise at an emotional level. For example, focusing on breathing might develop a state of gratitude, rather than one of presence, or joy. When focusing on breathing generates these emotions in you you feel them growing within the body and increasing. These distinctions about what everyone prefers to focus on are actually the different meditation techniques if you remember what we described in the section on the main techniques. For now let's keep it simple, just focus on the breath in the way that is easiest for you.

Surely, when you start concentrating only on your breath at some point different thoughts will start to cross your mind. Don't worry, this is normal, it happens to everyone all the time. It is difficult for people to stay focused only on one image or only on one thing. The mind is like that, we get distracted, other thoughts come across, or physical distractions interrupt our concentration. This causes us to lose the object of our focus, but you don't have to worry because that is part of the practice. What is important is to bring your attention back to the object of your focus as soon as you realize you have lost it. When you notice your distraction it means that you are well along in the process of learning meditation. You have noticed that your mind has left for other shores, that it has started building a movie, but you can come back from there and you can bring your mind where you want, and that is back to the object of your focus.

When you start meditating, especially the very first few times, you will not notice that you have lost your focus, or at any rate, you will notice very few times that the mind has become distracted. In those moments you are not meditating, in truth. With time and practice, you will notice more often the distractions of your mind and you will be quickly capable to go back with your focus to the object of your practice. You will even get to the point where you become less and less distracted throughout your practice and keep your focus and concentration longer and longer.

Well, let's put together the initial suggestions I've given you and create your first little meditation together.

1. Choose your position and sit down.

2. Close your eyes.

3. Take three deep breaths where you inhale through your nose and exhale through your mouth. Use these breaths to create space in your body and mind.

4. After the three deep breaths, you should start breathing only through your nose. The breath should flow easily and freely. Do not control it, do not modify it, just observe it. Observe every time the air comes in and every time the air goes out.

5. Visualize the air entering your nostrils when you inhale and leaving your nostrils when you exhale.

6. It may also help you to feel the sensations in your body, for example, your chest and navel expanding when you inhale and relaxing when you exhale.

7. If a thought comes to distract you, don't worry about it because it is part of meditation. Accept that it has come, let it go, and go back to focusing on the breath. Go back to feeling and listening to your breath.

8. Keep giving your full attention to your breath.

9. If again a distraction or a thought comes, let go. Don't judge yourself for being distracted. Just let go of the thought and bring your attention back to your breath.

10. Stay in meditation for as long as you like. Remember that even a few minutes may be enough at first (maybe 3 minutes or 5 minutes, then you can slowly increase).

11. When you feel ready to return, slowly start moving your fingers on your hands and move them for a few seconds.

12. Now take a deep breath, open your eyes and return to the reality around you.

13. Try to maintain the meditative state for a few seconds even with your eyes open in your surrounding reality so you will bring the positive feelings acquired with meditation into your day. Then get up, but only when you feel ready to do so.

Great! Very well done, you have just successfully completed your first meditation. I am sure it has gone very well. Keep practicing at least once a day and you will see that it will get better and easier every time. In the meantime, proceed with your reading to find out more information, tips, and techniques.

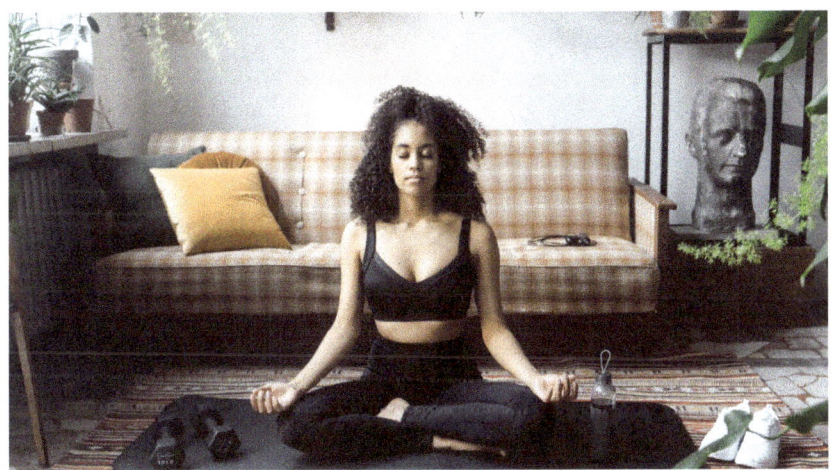

Meditation and Routine

Meditation must become your daily routine. Don't be frightened by my statement because it only takes very little time to achieve enormous benefits. When I say little time, I really mean it. Even a handful of minutes each day can be enough.

Don't imagine that you have to meditate for hours in the perfect lotus position. The important thing is to meditate daily and make meditation part of your daily routine. You don't even have to sit cross-legged on the floor. You can sit in a chair, lie on a cushion or a mat, whatever is best for you, as long as you meditate regularly and consistently for even a few minutes every day.

Nowadays, we all live extremely dynamic, often hectic lives. We are constantly inside our heads, always inside our whirling thoughts, busy doing a thousand things. We are caught up in the lives of other people we are somehow connected to and we interact with them constantly, either directly or perhaps through the various social media, on which we spend a significant amount of time during our days.

For all these reasons, meditation must your daily routine. Amid this chaos and frenzy, it is essential to stop for a moment of calm and peace and to find a moment entirely for yourself.

You need meditation in your routine to have a fixed moment each day in which you are sure to empty your mind and take care of yourself. Not only that, but you also need this moment to recharge your body and mind. Body and mind are deeply connected and to function well they need to be rebalanced, recharged, and reconnected at least once a day. Your daily meditation routine allows you to make all this happen.

You only need a few minutes to close your eyes and try to empty your mind, relax, and try to reach a state of peace. Try to find harmony, a sense of connection, and presence in the "here and now". This is very important, being in the present moment is essential and meditation allows you to achieve this condition.

To be in the present moment you need to turn your attention inward. The world we live in, however, always tries to make you do the opposite. We are always focused on the people around us, on what is going on around us, but not enough on what is going on inside us. Instead, it is so important to regularly take some time to go inside ourselves and be alone with ourselves for a little while.

As I told you, making meditation a small part of your daily routine is very important, but it is equally important to live this experience well. You must not see it as an imposition, nor as a complicated commitment. You must live it simply and lightly, as a small adventure within yourself, a great little journey of your own discovery. A journey within yourself that will bring you so many benefits.

Where to Meditate and How Long

The main purpose of meditation is to be able to concentrate and detach from external stimuli by turning the senses outward. That being said, what is the best place to meditate? The answer is simple and twofold.

The best place to meditate is where YOU can best put yourself in a position to concentrate and turn your senses inward. Having said that, however, I would tell you not to be too conditioned by the place otherwise you risk never meditating. If you get distracted at home, if at the office during your break is no good, you can't every day drop everything and take refuge in a Tibetan monastery to meditate. You have to create an ideal space for yourself where you can meditate daily and then when you can afford it, have a special experience by going to meditate in a special place if you feel the need or dream of having this experience.

Let's look at the main options available to you and the pros and cons of the various environments.

At Home

I would start with your home because it is the most practical place to meditate and the one in which you should feel most comfortable.

The main problem with home arises the moment you share it with someone, be it your family or a roommate. Someone might disturb you during meditation, so it would be ideal to let them know when not to disturb you.

My advice is to create a small meditation corner in your house and make it comfortable. Some small touches can create the atmosphere and facilitate concentration, for example, incense or essential oils, a soft and comfortable rug with your meditation cushion ready for you on it, and comfortable clothes waiting in your corner to wrap you in comfort. In short, there are really so many possibilities, some even with therapeutic purposes, for example, to unblock the Chakras. If this topic interests you, you will find lots of detailed information in my book "Chakras for Beginners," where there is an extensive section on meditation for the Chakras and how to create the ideal meditation corner.

The advantages of this solution are quite obvious. It is a free and practical solution, in fact, you will not have to incur additional expenses, you will not have time constraints, and you will not have to move around to meditate. The disadvantage is the distraction it can represent, both if you live with others who can be a distraction for you, and because the environment itself can distract you by being full of personal stimuli.

Outdoors

There are so many options for meditating outdoors, of course, conditioned by where you live, but let's say there are a few for everyone. Contact with nature helps a lot to get into a meditative state, so this is a very good option, but temperature and weather conditions have to be taken into account.

Let's say that in nice weather or warm weather meditating outdoors is really a worthwhile experience. I suffer a lot from the cold, so for me, this practice is not good if I am in a cold season or place, however it might be good for those who do not suffer from the cold or live in a warm place all year round.

If you live in the city, you can find a space to meditate in a park or public garden. If you live in the country, you could have your own private garden or unearth some other delightful corner in nature. If you live by the sea or in the mountains, you are very lucky. You enjoy the energy of two very powerful elements from which your meditation will benefit enormously, and besides, there will be plenty of quiet and beautiful places to choose from.

Since you need to focus and turn your gaze inward, I recommend that you take 3 elements into account when choosing your temple in nature:

1. Choose a place that is not crowded, so as not to be disturbed and distracted

2. Choose a place that is not a point of transit, for the same reasons

3. Choose a place where it is easy to sit. If you sit on the floor, you need to be able to get up and sit nimbly and comfortably. Otherwise, you might have to opt for a bench, using the position described for chair meditation in the chapter "How to Start Meditating"

Again, the pros are convenience and low cost. If you choose a place close enough to home, the cost of getting there will be very limited and you will not have any particular time constraints. On the other hand, what will constrain you will be the weather, temperatures, and possible intruders to distract you if you have not chosen a secluded enough place.

Meditation Schools or Specialized Centers

This option is more for those who live in cities large enough to accommodate these kinds of facilities, which, although they are spreading widely, are still not available in many of the smaller towns.

In these facilities, it is always possible to avail yourself of a teacher to support you on the path, although, in my opinion, learning to meditate is a very intimate, personal, and individual path that you may want to take alone.

In this circumstance advantages and disadvantages have to be calculated on a more personal level. The possibility of having a teacher for some might be an advantage. Another advantage for some might be that you need an appointment to attend these facilities, and this can help in maintaining a commitment to meditate and regularity in doing so. For those a bit more creative this could, however, be a disadvantage, forcing an act that should be more spontaneous. This submission to schedules would make a spiritual practice that should not be so too mechanical.

Moreover, here it is a matter of adapting to these centers' schedules and not one's own, and this can complicate matters for those whose lifestyles are constrained by rhythms and thighs schedules. Finally, these facilities are fee-based, certainly with options for all budgets, but for many, this can be a drawback.

Special Locations

As I mentioned at the beginning of this chapter, the choice of these special, mystical locations is not about daily meditation. The choice should fall on these special locations when you feel you need a break from daily life when you need to disconnect from your daily routine to immerse yourself in another dimension. The beneficial effect on you is indescribable and it is an experience that I would highly recommend as you begin to gain experience in the practice of meditation.

There are many special locations you can choose from, everywhere around the world, depending on your budget and how far you want to travel.

There are many farmhouses equipped as a place of refuge from everyday life where you can go to meditate. In these facilities, you can immerse yourself in meditation in close contact with wonderful nature as your backdrop.

Other options are monasteries or ashrams. Both of these facilities can be found anywhere in the world, it is up to you to decide whether you want to travel all the way to India or if you prefer one near your city, a choice that also depends on the kind of experience you want to have. I think the concept of a monastery is familiar to pretty much everyone, I mean the place where monks live and pray. The Ashram, on the other hand, is a physical place where you can devote yourself to meditation and prayer, a well-defined place that has this specific purpose. Its name comes from the Indian term "ashrama," which means "place of rest." These are silent places, in close contact with nature, where one goes in search of self through a spiritual path. One meditates, practices the discipline of yoga, studies traditional sacred texts, prays, and travels in search of one's essence through these mystical practices.

The downside of these options, as I mentioned earlier, is that you risk making your meditation practice an occasional factor related to your stay in these facilities. It is self-evident that you cannot attend them daily, and if you only meditate in these places you would find yourself meditating a handful of times a year at best.

If, on the other hand, staying in these facilities becomes an extra to your daily meditation routine, these experiences immediately become a benefit of enormous proportions. They will exponentially improve the quality of your life, accentuating the benefits given by your daily meditation. In addition, the change of experience and setting will help you ensure that meditation remains a spontaneous and deeply spiritual experience, and does not just become a mechanical, forced, and unfelt habit.

Now that we have extensively discussed where to meditate, let's talk about how long you should meditate.

So, "How long should I meditate?" I would say that this question falls into the top 5 that I receive most frequently. The other 4 you can guess because I have answered them in previous chapters. What is meditation? What is it for? How do I start meditating? What technique do I choose? Where do I meditate? For how long?

The answer is, "It depends…"

Let's start with the premise that mediation is an appointment with yourself and must first and foremost be a pleasant time and not an obligation. That is why I say "It depends…," because the right time is the one that gives pleasure to you.

Another consideration we encountered earlier is that it is better to meditate a little, but constantly, than a lot, but sporadically.

Finally, there is the consideration that the depth of meditation matters much more than its duration.

That being said, I reiterate what I said in the chapter on how to start meditating. It only takes a few minutes a day, once or several times a day depending on how you feel, possibly making it a daily appointment, a routine, for you.

You can start with a few minutes the first week (1 to 3 minutes), then increase to 5 minutes the second week. You can choose to do it once a day, at a specific time of the day that suits you best, or several times a day. For example, 5 minutes in the morning to get your day off to a good start, 5 minutes in the afternoon to dissipate stress as it builds up, and 5 minutes in the evening to relax before bedtime.

In subsequent weeks, you might gradually increase to 10 minutes, then 20, then half an hour. Many even go up to an hour. Don't let these time slots make you feel uncomfortable. I reiterate the concept that the right time is the right time for you. However, I can tell you, with deep awareness, that everyone who starts on the path of meditation, as soon as they begin to enjoy the benefits and see the first improvements in their lives, want more, and this brings with it the desire, willingness and desire to extend the meditation time.

So start with a few minutes, try to be consistent, learn to go deep and listen to yourself, meditate for as long as you feel like doing it, and whenever you feel the need for its benefits.

What has been said so far applies to daily meditations. If you go to a monastery or other places of retreat to disconnect from the stress of the world around you, in that case, you have different needs, for longer and deeper meditations probably. Make the most of those experiences to embark on a wonderful journey within yourself.

I would like to end this chapter with a little advice that comes from direct and personal experience. Often during the day, you happen to feel upset because of some events or situations that have happened, other times you feel nervous and insecure about an important event. In all circumstances of discomfort, going for a minute to a quiet corner for a mini-meditation can totally change the fortunes of a day. You really just need a tiny bit of time. Sit down if you can, close your eyes, breathe deeply and consciously, focus your attention on your breath, calm your thoughts and turn to your inner self. That's all it really takes, just a minute or two to eliminate anxiety, stress, insecurity, and other discomforts. You will feel better because of that single minute of meditation, you will be more balanced, calm, centered, focused, and confident.

Breathing and Meditation

Another question I get asked very often is, "What is the right way to breathe during meditation?"

This is a very important question and deserves a detailed answer.

Breathing and meditation are deeply connected to each other. The goal of meditation is to slow down mental activity and we use breathing to achieve this goal. Through breathing, we try to quiet the mind and bring forth inner peace.

The best way to breathe during meditation is to breathe naturally through the nose. Breathing should not be intentionally altered; it should be allowed to flow spontaneously. You must concentrate on the sensation of the air entering and leaving your nostrils and become aware of this process. You have to bring all your attention to this awareness, focus on it, and exclude everything else around you.

As I already mentioned in the chapter on how to start meditating, at first your mind will be crowded with thoughts coming in and making it restless. The more stressed your mind is, the more thoughts will come crowding it as you enter the meditation state. You must let go of these thoughts; you must not follow them even though you will be tempted to do so. You must bring your attention and concentration back to your breath. As soon as your mind wanders off you bring it back to the breath. You will become better and better at doing this through consistent practice.

Remember to keep your breathing natural and fluid, do not alter it, or breathe intentionally. When you breathe naturally, every time you throw out air there is a small pause that is completely natural. It is important not to interrupt this little pause by intentionally altering your breathing because the interruption would cause you to gasp.

The inhalation phase is the phase in which thoughts move and agitate; during the small pause after exhalation, you feel the sense of calmness reverberating in your mind. You must try to take advantage of this calmness to quiet your thoughts before the new inhalation phase. Try to avoid the feeling of numbness that will develop in you during that small pause because that is what makes many people fall asleep when they meditate. Treasure this advice because so many people tell me that they fall asleep when they try to meditate.

There are some meditation techniques with specific purposes where you have to learn to control your breathing consciously. By consciously controlling your breath you can alter your mental patterns, you can calm the mind, make it clearer and more rational to make better decisions, and better manage emotions, especially negative ones. By consciously controlling your breath you can improve sleep quality, concentration level, and memory abilities. Thus, by changing the way you breathe during your meditation, you can change situations and conditions in your daily life. For example, you can better manage emotions, solve insomnia problems, concentration problems, memory problems, and much more.

I would like to share some information that is easy to understand, but a little bit more advanced. For someone, it will be useful for knowledge, while for someone else it will be a useful exercise to take a step forward after the first few weeks of practicing traditional meditation.

In the chapter on meditation techniques, we talked about "Intentional Meditation." Now, I would like to share with you some controlled breathing techniques with specific purposes that you can practice precisely during intentional meditation sessions.

Ujjayi breathing

The term "Ujjayi" comes from Sanskrit and literally means "victory," so Ujjayi breathing is translated as "victorious breath."

It is called this way because its proper practice allows one to calm the mind and be in the "here and now," so this breathing technique "wins" the mind, and controls it by quieting it and making it present. It is the breathing technique performed during yoga and if you are a partitioner you may be familiar with it.

The intentional reasons for its practice during meditation are many and reflect the countless benefits it brings to the quality of our lives. As I have said it calms the mind and gives awareness. In addition, calming the mind reduces stress and nervous tension. By inducing this state of deep relaxation, it is also very helpful against insomnia. It is an excellent tool for deepening the connection between body, mind, and spirit.

How to practice it:

1. Sit in a comfortable position, with your back straight, but not stiff, and your neck and shoulders relaxed. Use a pillow if you sit on the floor. Rest your hands on your thighs or knees. (Go review the chapter "How to start meditating" if you have doubts).

2. Close your eyes, and take three deep breaths inhaling through your nose and exhaling through your mouth. Then breathe in through your nose only and begin to focus on controlling your breathing.

3. Breathing through the nose should be in one smooth, deep flow. Inhalation and exhalation should be the same duration, about 4 seconds each is fine. Count the duration of the first few breaths to gain awareness of the length of inhalation and exhalation.

4. The key part of this technique, however, is that you have to make the temperate of your breath a lot warmer. To do so you must, still keeping your mouth closed and your jaw relaxed, contract the glottis and let the air pass through it producing a sound that resembles an aspirated H. (It resembles the sound you make with your mouth when you breathe on the glass to mist it, but you have to do it with your nose.) The air will make contact with the glottis and the blood vessels will make this air very warm.

5. You will need to hear the sound of your breath throughout the meditation, and you will need to hear it (and thus produce it) on both inhalation and exhalation. Be careful not to close the glottis too much because you

will block the passage of air. The closure should be the minimum necessary to produce the desired sound.

6. Throughout the meditation you should focus on keeping your breathing deliberate, controlled, and steady (4 seconds inhalation and 4 seconds exhalation. You can make 3 seconds and 3 seconds if 4 is too long for you). Go deeper and deeper while maintaining a steady flow and concentration on breath control. Turn all your attention inward with your mind-calming, relaxing, and letting go of all thoughts except breath control.

7. Meditate for as long as you feel. When you decide to stop, bring your breathing back to natural, always from the nose though. Start moving your fingers to slowly return to the world around you, and open your eyes only when you feel ready.

TIP: To tell if you are performing this breathing technique correctly listen to your body. If your chest expands and your abdomen contracts, you are breathing correctly.

Kapalabhati Breathing

The name of this technique comes from Sanskrit and is translated as "Breath of Fire."

It is an energizing breathing technique. With this technique you oxygenate the body and receive three main beneficial effects:

- It improves concentration

- It eliminates feelings of sleepiness and exhaustion

- It fills the body with revitalizing energy

How to practice it:

1. Sit in a comfortable position, with your back straight, but not stiff, and your neck and shoulders relaxed. Use a pillow if you sit on the floor. Rest your hands on your thighs or knees. (Go review the chapter "How to start meditating" if you have doubts).

2. Close your eyes, and take three deep breaths inhaling through your nose and exhaling through your mouth. Then breathe in through your nose only and begin to focus on controlling your breathing.

3. Breathe in as deeply as you can, expanding your abdomen as you do so.

4. Now you must exhale all the air at once, and to do this you must contract your abdominal muscles abruptly and forcefully.

5. Continue with these strong, short breaths and you will begin to feel a warm sensation in the abdominal area. Remember that the abdomen should be relaxed when you inhale and contracted only when you exhale.

6. Meditate for as long as you feel is good for you, although 3 groups of 15 breaths each are recommended for this breathing technique. A full breath is composed of inhalation and exhalation. After 15 full breaths, take a short break and then resume with another cycle of 15 breaths.

7. When you decide to stop, return your breathing to its natural flow, always through the nose though. Start moving your fingers to slowly return to the world around you, and open your eyes only when you feel ready.

Relaxation Breathing

As you can easily deduce from the name, this breathing technique aims to relax and unwind.

The main benefits of this technique are closely related to the state of relaxation in which it places you. Your mind will be free from anxiety and stress, and this condition will also help you sleep better.

How to practice it:

1. Lie down facing up. A gym mat or yoga mat is fine. The important thing is that you are lying on a comfortable surface without anything hurting or bothering you. Extend your arms along your sides with your palms facing upward. If you practice yoga or are familiar with the main postures, this breathing is practiced in the Savasana posture.

2. Get comfortable in the position, close your eyes, and breathe through your nose. Release your mind, focus on your breathing, and on controlling it.

3. Inhale the airflow for 3 seconds and exhale for 6 seconds (you can mentally count to get the rhythm of breathing). Exhaling twice as long as inhaling puts into action the mechanism our body has for relaxing. You should leave a small pause, even just a couple of seconds, between the exhalation and the new inhalation to make the technique even more effective.

4. Meditate and breathe for as long as you need to. Ideally, you should continue until your body and mind are both in a state of total calm, peace, and relaxation.

5. When you decide to stop, bring your breathing back to its natural flow, always from the nose though. Start moving

your fingers to slowly return to the world around you and open your eyes only when you feel ready.

Diaphragmatic Breathing

Its name comes from the part of your body mainly involved in this technique.

Practicing this breathing technique allows you to enter a state of well-being that helps you quickly eliminate stress and is an extremely useful technique for controlling your emotional states.

How to practice it:

1. Lie down facing up. A gym mat or yoga mat is fine. The important thing is that you are lying on a comfortable surface without anything hurting or bothering you. Bend your legs with your feet about 8 inches apart. Place one hand with the palm on your chest and one hand with the palm on your belly. The hands allow you to feel your diaphragm.

2. Get comfortable in the position, close your eyes, and breathe through your nose. Release the mind, focus on your breathing, and on controlling it.

3. Bring your attention to your belly. Breathe in deeply through your nose and let the air go into your belly. Then slowly exhale. It would be ideal to exhale through your nose. If at first attempts, you just can't do it, you can exhale through your mouth, but your goal should be to complete the whole breath properly through the nose. Exhale naturally, without forcing the air out. The purpose of the hand on your chest is to make sure that this does not rise. Instead, you need to feel the belly rise and the hand resting on it will allow you to do this.

4. Meditate and breathe for as long as you feel necessary. When you decide to stop, bring your breathing back to its natural flow, always from the nose though. Start moving the fingers of your hands to slowly return to the world around you and open your eyes only when you feel ready.

TIP: To tell if you are practicing correctly you should have the hand on your chest completely still both when you inhale and when you exhale. The one on your belly, on the other hand, should move and follow the movement of your breath by rising and falling. If the hand on your chest rises, it means you are not using your diaphragm to breathe and you need to try again and practice.

Calming Breathing

Some call this technique the "4 7 8 Breathing". The first name comes from the state it allows you to reach, while the second comes from the breathing times to practice it, which I will explain in a moment.

How to practice it:

1. Sit in a comfortable position, with your back straight, but not stiff, and your neck and shoulders relaxed. Use a pillow if you sit on the floor. Rest your hands on your thighs or knees. (Go review the chapter "How to start meditating" if you have doubts).

2. Close your eyes, and take three deep breaths inhaling through your nose and exhaling through your mouth. Then breathe in through your nose only and start focusing on controlling your breathing.

3. Breathe in for 4 seconds. Hold your breath for 7 seconds. Exhale for 8 seconds. Repeat the cycle.

4. Meditate and breathe for as long as you feel necessary. When you decide to stop, return your breathing to its natural flow, always through the nose though. Start moving your fingers to slowly return to the world around you and open your eyes only when you feel ready.

Breathing for Positivity

Some call this technique the "3 5 3 Breathing". The first name comes from what it enables you to achieve and the second from the breathing times to practice it, which I will explain in a moment.

The main purpose of this technique is to expel all negative energies from the body to remain pervaded by positive ones. As the oxygen circulates, it will cleanse your energy, eliminating anxiety and negativity, and leaving you present, centered, and focused.

How to practice it:

1. Sit in a comfortable position, with your back straight, but not stiff, and your neck and shoulders relaxed. Use a pillow if you sit on the floor. Rest your hands on your thighs or knees. (Go review the chapter "How to start meditating" if you have doubts).

2. Close your eyes, and take three deep breaths inhaling through your nose and exhaling through your mouth. Then breathe in through your nose only and start focusing on controlling your breathing.

3. Breathe in for 3 seconds. Hold your breath for 5 seconds. Exhale for 3 seconds. Repeat the cycle.

4. Meditate and breathe for as long as you feel necessary. When you decide to stop, return your breathing to its natural flow, always through the nose though. Start moving your fingers to slowly return to the world around you and open your eyes only when you feel ready.

Before I conclude the chapter on breathing there are a couple of points I would like to bring to your attention. First, you may have noticed that throughout this section, and in the book in general, I always emphasize that you have to breathe through your nose. This is not accidental. On the contrary, it is not only important but fundamental.

Only by breathing through the nose can our body control the perfect and optimal intake of CO_2 and release NO, which strengthens the immune system, stimulates blood circulation, and helps sexuality. When you breathe through your mouth you expel too much CO_2.

When air passes through the nostrils it is filtered of impurities and is, therefore, of better quality than air inhaled through the mouth, which does not have this filtering function. The nose also warms the air and humidifies it before it enters our internal organs. The mouth cannot perform these two functions either. Therefore, when you breathe through your mouth, you are putting too dry air into your organs and, often, that air is also too cold compared to the ideal temperature of that organ, which will consume your energy to bring the air temperature up to its ideal standard.

Breathing well and consciously can therefore bring so many benefits to your well-being, not only on a physical level.

Our breathing influences our emotional state too and, on the other hand, our emotional state controls our breathing. This is why breathing well and knowing how to control your breathing are so important for your well-being. If you are breathing laboredly, you will find yourself in a state of anxiety and stress. If you are anxious and stressed your breathing will be quite labored. I am sure you have noticed it before.

So, I recommend analyzing your breathing, just because breathing is natural does not mean you are doing it correctly. Throughout your life, you may have picked up bad breathing habits without even realizing it. Use what you have learned in this chapter to do a little analysis. Then use meditation to practice a better kind of breathing. Slowly start using the techniques you have learned to improve the way you breathe throughout your day. You will gain huge benefits by simply breathing better during your day.

You may have noticed that in the chapter on "How to Start Meditating" in step 3 (and also in this chapter) I wrote about taking 3 deep breaths, inhaling through the nose, and exhaling through the mouth. This is one of the rare cases where I recommend mouth breathing, but there is a reason. Exhaling through the mouth is very useful in times of anxiety, stress, and nervousness because it helps release the tension that pervades you. I find it a useful practice for beginners in meditation because they are often a bit tense from facing something new and many times they have accumulated and never discharged tensions that complicate their first approaches to the new practice.

Another circumstance that I frequently notice in those who have never meditated or approached disciplines such as yoga and some martial arts is that they breathe mostly through their mouths and approaching breathing only through their noses seems difficult for them, almost as if they are not getting enough air into their bodies. The way they breathe is mainly a habit, I have already explained why nasal breathing is the most correct. I would like to give a few small suggestions to override the habit of mouth breathing and start breathing mainly through the nose, in case you are part of this group of people.

First, throughout the day try to keep your mouth closed as much as possible, this will somehow prompt you to make more use of your nose. There are several nasal breathing exercises. I feel like recommending one in particular to you, both to strengthen the use of the nose in breathing and to make sure that the nostrils are free and always working at their best.

Alternate Nostril Breathing

When we breathe through our nose to us it seems that we are always using both nostrils, but in fact, we are not. It is a completely natural process; our body chooses to use only one nostril rather than another. It usually chooses to use for breathing the one opposite the half of the brain that is doing most of the work at that given moment.

The benefits this exercise brings are many. As mentioned earlier, it allows the nostrils to be kept wide open at all times, if practiced regularly. It also creates a profound balance between mind and body and is therefore great for keeping nervousness away and staving off the onset of anxiety.

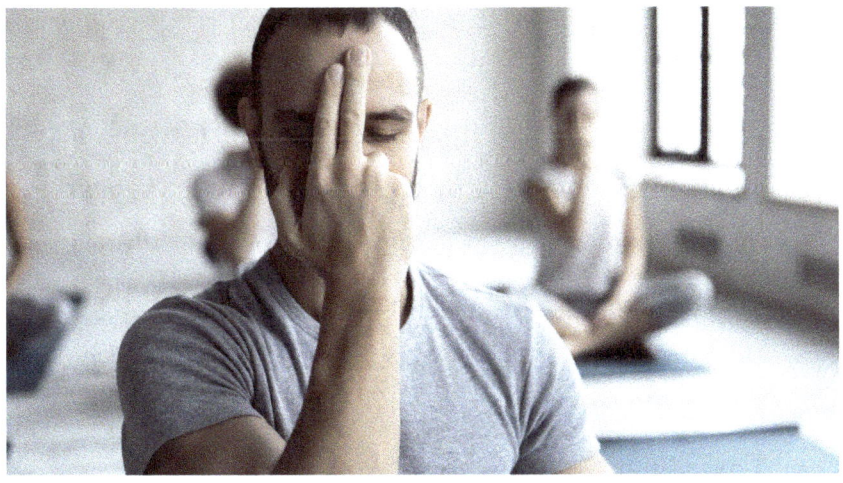

How to practice it:

1. Sit in a comfortable position, with your back straight, but not stiff, and your neck and shoulders relaxed. Use a pillow if you sit on the floor. Rest your right hand on your thigh or knee. Rest the index and middle fingers of your left hand in the space between your eyebrows.

2. With your thumb close the left nostril. Exhale the air already foraged through the right nostril and then inhale again through the right nostril.

3. Remove thumb pressure and clear the left nostril and close the right nostril with the ring finger and little finger. Exhale through the left nostril and then inhale again through the left nostril.

4. Move your fingers as described above and exhale from the right nostril.

5. What is described in the previous points is a complete breathing cycle with this technique. Practice repeating the cycle several times for a few minutes, 15 times is a good repetition time. Remember to complete the exercise by exhaling through the right nostril.

Well done! You now have a great deal of useful information about breathing. All you have to do is put it into practice in conjunction with your meditation sessions to enjoy the immense benefits that both practices can bring to your life.

What Do You Need to Meditate?

I am often asked if anything, in particular, is needed to meditate. No, you do not need anything special to meditate; in fact, you can meditate by simply sitting in a chair.

However, various gadgets can make your meditation more comfortable, especially if you decide to meditate sitting on the floor in the classic meditation position (which is called Sukhasana, meaning "comfortable position").

1. The Mat

The first thing that comes to my mind is the mat. I am referring to gym mats, those commonly used for doing yoga are a perfect solution. They give some comfort and softness. If you meditate outdoors they prevent you from getting dirty, feeling the dampness off the ground and its eventual roughness.

This is especially true for beginners. With time you may begin to appreciate meditating outdoors in direct contact with the earth. It is a wonderful experience feeling the Earth's energy flowing directly into you, without interference. Feeling the warm sand beneath you, the earth between the roots of a tree, or the grass of a meadow is great, but for those who are just starting out it is a bit uncomfortable because you are not yet trained or used to it, so you might find a mat useful at least at the beginning.

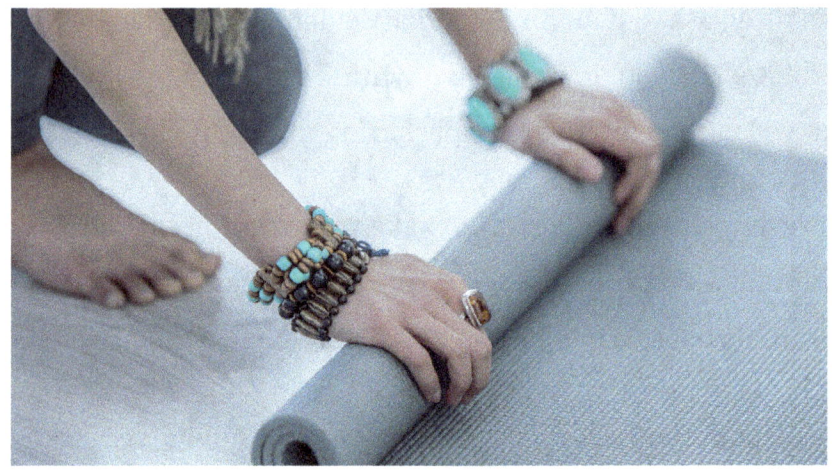

2. Meditation Pillows

You can find them in many shapes, materials, and sizes. They all have the same function of making you feel comfortable during your meditation. I mentioned their use in the chapter on "How to start meditating", and to choose the most appropriate one, you need to figure out what position you are most comfortable sitting in.

Especially in the beginning, using a cushion is always recommended. Your body is not yet trained and accustomed to holding the Sukhasana position or even sitting with your back straight for too long. Therefore, without the help of a cushion, your back may hurt, or the part you are sitting on may be sore because the mat is not thick enough. Conditions of pain or lack of comfort would put your body in such a tense state that it would become an obstacle making your practice more difficult to perform, which is why you might need a good cushion to start with. Over time you may no longer feel the need for it, although this certainly depends a lot on age and physical condition.

Of course, you can also use a pillow you already have, perhaps folding it up or otherwise adapting it to your need.

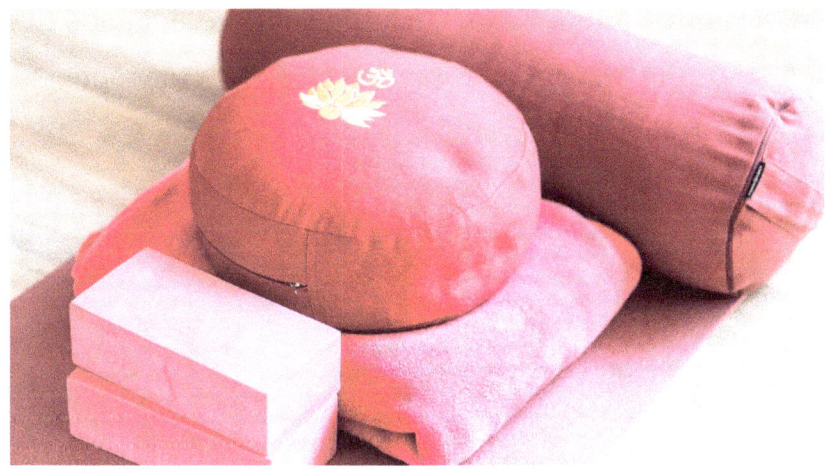

3. Comfortable Clothing

Practicing wearing soft clothing that does not compress and oppress you is a huge benefit to your practice because it is easier to relax while wearing comfortable clothing.

If you meditate indoors you can certainly equip yourself with whatever makes you feel most comfortable, if you meditate outdoors you might consider an outfit that is comfortable but does not make you feel uneasy if you were to meet other people.

If you meditate in the office, you don't need to change, but it might be very helpful to take off your jacket, loosen your belt, undo the button on your pants, take off your tie, and undo the first few buttons on your shirt (and for ladies it's the same, try to get rid of too oppressive restraints) and so on.

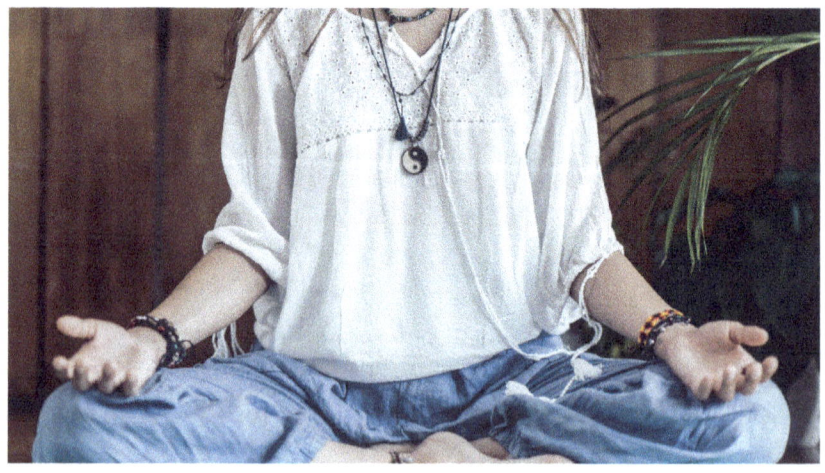

4. Furnishing

This covers a more advanced stage, but it is worth mentioning. If meditation becomes an integral part of your life, as I firmly believe it will, at some point you will feel the need to carve out a little corner of your home that will become your own little sanctuary, your own meditation corner.

You will certainly want to furnish it in some way and decorate it so that it will be even more personal, so that it will be pervaded with energy, and you will just walk into it to feel better and leave out all the ugliness of your day. I'll tell you a little bit about mine to give you an idea, and if you want to go deeper, as I already told you, in my book "Chakras for Beginners" you can find a lot of useful information. I put soft mats on the floor with the colors of the Chakra energy. I scattered the mats with colorful pillows, again to encourage the energy. I added a very low wooden coffee table on which there is an incense burner in which I burn different incense according to the energy I want to stimulate, stones and crystals for all 7 Chakras also lay on that table so that they pervade my energy corner, and last there is a small speaker that I use to broadcast the sounds of nature or to play relaxing music or guided meditations.

Lighting is also very important. In this case, there are mainly three options. You could choose an adjustable intensity lamp placed in a corner and set it to a different intensity according to your needs. You could use candles to set the mood. Finally, you could opt for a Himalayan salt lamp that gives off a warm, soft light with a strong emotional impact. Here the choice is really yours. I can tell you that I do some of my mentor's guided meditations in total darkness, wearing an airplane mask to cover any source of light, but in most cases, I prefer a soft light with warm tones.

In your corner, you might want to put curtains, and sofa covers, you might prefer an essential oil diffuser instead of incense, and you might choose a salt lamp rather than candles. The important thing is that the place reflects your personality and your taste, makes you feel good and gives you the energies and the emotions you need.

Many people find it unnecessary to create this corner because they prefer to meditate outdoors, and the impact of nature infuses them with the same energy. I have found it essential because living in a big northern city, the weather has often been a hindrance, as has contact with nature, which can be reached in rather long spaces of time if you are not lucky enough to live near a decent park to go and practice in. So, consider investing some time and a little money in creating your own little corner of the world. If you are also as creative as I am, you will find it an enjoyable, fun, and ever-evolving activity. Your space will evolve with you, reflect your changes, and always make you feel good.

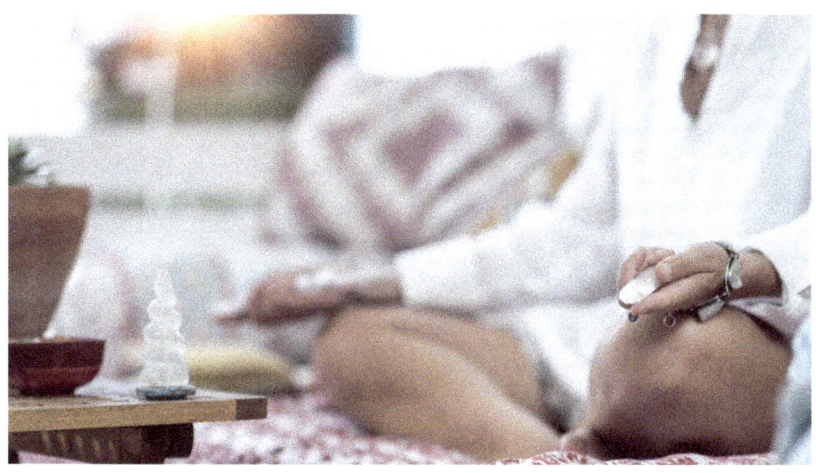

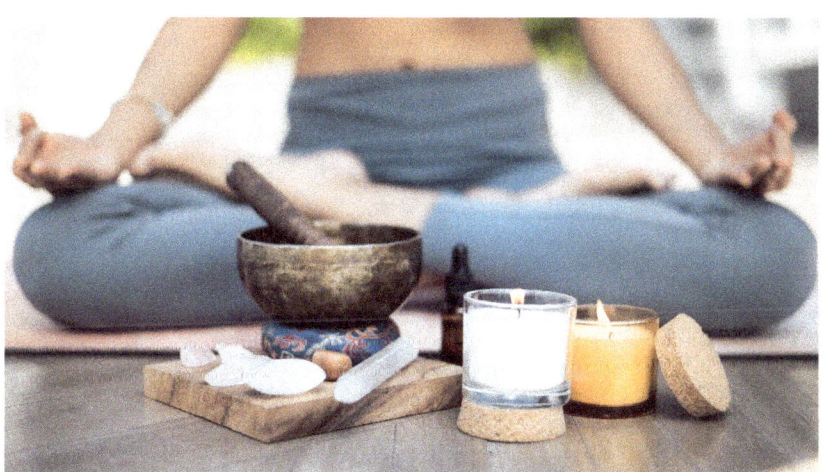

The 9 Benefits of Meditation

The benefits of meditation are measured through the positive changes that occur in your daily life. The happier you feel and the more you feel in control of your life, the more effect meditation is having on your daily life.

The purpose of meditation is to make you a better version of yourself and it does this by helping you to eliminate old, narrow mental patterns and limiting habits. With constant meditation, you will create habits and mental patterns that are much more positive and functional for living a wonderful life. You will gradually see this wonder unfold like a small miracle in all aspects of your life.

Meditation allows you to feel better mentally and emotionally, and this has a huge reflection on your physical well-being. If you are well emotionally and mentally, these two factors will not weigh on the health of your body and you will feel better in general. It is easier to get sick for those people who have emotional or mental problems and, in fact, this category of people is always plagued by a thousand aches and pains. Meditation can help you get out of this loop.

Let's see together what are the main benefits that each of us can gain by consistently meditating for at least a few minutes a day.

1. Meditation Reduces Stress

Many medical studies have shown that meditation is an excellent tool for reducing symptoms given by stress.

Stress is given by the increase in our bodies of cortisol, a hormone that is also commonly referred to as "the stress hormone." When levels of this hormone in our bodies rise we feel stressed mentally and physically. Cortisol creates the release of inflammatory substances that have a whole range of repercussions on our bodies.

Stress tends to create states of anxiety and depression, deteriorates the quality of sleep, causes fatigue, makes your thinking lose clarity, and can cause high blood pressure.

Being able to reduce stress through the practice of meditation can bring enormous benefits to the practitioner's life, reducing the risk of incurring all these uncomfortable states.

2. Meditation Helps Control Anxiety

There are an increasing number of medical studies conducted on people who regularly practice meditation that prove the deep benefits you can gain.

Numerous studies have shown that those who regularly practice meditation tend not to be plagued by anxiety or, at any rate, can control it much better and not be overwhelmed by it.

Meditation is, in fact, a very useful exercise to combine with the various medical therapies given by doctors to patients to manage social anxiety or panic attacks.

If you work in a very competitive environment it can help you relieve the anxiety and stress of everyday situations.

By reducing anxiety, you also reduce the possibility of becoming involved in diseases that arise from anxiety and its various side effects.

3. Meditation Helps Manage Emotions

Meditation can be used to create emotions and feelings other than those we experience. If you are plagued by negative feelings and emotions, which tend to make you feel depressed, meditation allows you to create positive feelings. With these new positive feelings you can, then, create a more positive overall outlook and positive habits, to live life more peacefully. You also learn, in this way, how to deal with painful events and live at peace with yourself and the world.

4. Meditation Gives You Awareness

As I mentioned in the introductory part of this chapter, meditation allows you to become the best version of yourself.

As you get to know yourself better and on a deeper and more intimate level, you become more aware of yourself. This awareness leads you to be better with yourself, but also to relate better to others and to the world around you. You will be better off in your life because you will have healthier relationships with those around you, and with yourself, and solving problems will become easier.

Through meditation, you will be able to identify harmful thoughts and bad, weakening thought habits. Only by knowing these negative points, can you take action on them and turn them into positives.

5. Meditation Makes You More Mindful

When you meditate and bring all your attention to the breath, mantras, sensations, emotions, or whatever the object of your meditation is, and you learn over time to keep this attention longer and longer, you generate tremendous benefit in your daily life as well.

This ability that you learn and improve during meditation to maintain attention for longer and longer times also occurs in your daily life.

Several scientific tests have been done on this benefit, from which it was found that those who practice meditation on a sustained and consistent basis can maintain attention at high levels for longer, without getting tired even in stressful situations, than those who do not practice meditation. The test was done in highly competitive work environments and those who meditated managed to stay focused and undistracted for longer times than their colleagues who did not practice the discipline.

It emerged from this test that repeated practice of meditation reverses patterns of brain functioning that cause a lack of attention and the mind's tendency to wander, thus leading those patterns to work based on attention and focus.

This also leads to a decrease in worries because the brain is focused on what you choose and not wandering around getting lost in creating negative scenarios that will probably never come true, as often happens to those whose minds have a great tendency to wander. You exercise healthy control over your thought patterns and learn to redirect your thoughts positively.

6. Meditation Improves Your Memory

Because of the important improvement in attention that meditation gives you, you also gain a strong mental clarity that exerts a beneficial effect on the quality of your memory.

A clearer mind helps you remember things better. It also helps you keep your mind younger, preventing the effects of aging from occurring too soon and, in many cases, delaying them.

7. Meditation Makes You Sleep Better

As I mentioned in the conclusion of the fifth benefit, through meditation you learn to redirect your thoughts, thus moving the mind away from negative ones and toward positive ones.

Often insomnia, or at any rate poor sleep quality, is attributable to the thoughts we allow to haunt our minds. By being able to redirect these harmful thoughts you will be able to improve sleep quality.

According to scientific experiments on sleep quality, those who meditate fall asleep earlier and sleep longer and deeper.

However, it is not just a matter of thoughts. When you meditate you learn to let go of tension and relax your body and mind. These skills are very useful to fall asleep faster, and the sense of peace that accompanies meditation makes you sleep better and longer.

8. Meditation Makes you Become Kinder

As mentioned in several of the benefits listed in this chapter, meditation helps you positively redirect your thoughts. It also allows you to go very deep within yourself. In this way, you can generate deep, positive feelings toward yourself and then expand them to other people in your world.

You develop love and kindness toward yourself, and you can also share these feelings with those around you. This helps you feel more comfortable in a social group, not feel anxiety from contact with others, and manage anger better. The combination of these benefits helps you deal with difficult relationships with your partner, conflict marriages, or complicated family situations because you develop empathy, positivity, love, and kindness.

9. Meditation Helps You Fight Bad Habits

Daily behaviors and actions are 95% dictated by your habits. Often, you fail to achieve your goals in life because you have some bad habits that hinder you. Changing habits is a process that requires hard work, which is well rewarded by the benefits you gain. However, meditation tends to make this process much easier.

First, meditation helps you develop self-control and self-awareness, which are key elements in changing your habits for the better. Then, through meditation, you can direct impulses, emotions, and attention where you want, being able to understand why you behave in a certain way. In this way, you develop the willpower to correct that wrong habit that is hindering your success in any field.

The examples of hindering habits are so many and in so many areas. Think of someone who is looking for love but cannot stay faithful. Think about someone who wants a fabulous body but can't quench the nervous hunger. Think about someone who wants to have more money but spends more than he earns each month. Really, meditation can bring improvement and well-being in all areas of your life, at the cost of a handful of daily minutes that you can take away from useless activities, like watching TV.

Tips for Getting Started with Meditation

Start with a little. When you want to turn a practice into a habit, you have to start with little, but consistently, every day. Don't start with half an hour, but with a maximum of 5 or 10 minutes, possibly every day, as often as possible anyway.

Make it easy. Don't try a thousand meditation techniques, a hundred apps on your smartphone, and listen to ten different teachers. That would certainly complicate things for you. Try maybe two or three techniques, select a couple of apps to try, or pick a master or two to follow. Then figure out which technique you feel most comfortable with and focus on that. I recommend picking one or two at most to start with.

Schedule your meditation. Decide on a time and, if necessary, set the reminder via an alarm clock on your smartphone so you don't forget. It will seem a bit forced and lacking spontaneity at first, but it is not easy to develop new habits and you need to take advantage of all the tools you can to do so. Of course, on the other hand, you should not experience it as an unpleasant obligation. When the phone rings you should not be annoyed at the reminder but happy that it is time to meditate, a time to devote to yourself and your well-being. The purpose of scheduling meditation is to make the appointment with yourself as welcome and natural a habit as eating, showering, or dressing. You always find time to eat, shower, or dress in the morning. Similarly, it will have to be for meditation, another of the basic and indispensable elements for the well-being of your life.

Keep realistic expectations. You are a lot of conversations around you about meditation, and with all this talk you end up setting unrealistic expectations. Many people expect to receive enlightenment as soon as they start practicing. The first benefit you will get is to feel well, which seems to be an incredible accomplishment in a society where stress, anxiety, and emotional distress are always around the corner waiting for us. So, think about those realistic expectations when you decide to start to meditate. First of all the expectation of feeling well and continuing to get better and better. With time and practice, there will also be room for great revelations.

By meditating with the idea of doing good for yourself and experiencing meditation as taking time just for yourself, you will begin to make a very deep connection with yourself and begin to see the first immediate results in your outer world. You will begin to react differently to situations and circumstances, and you will relate differently to people in your personal life, but also in your professional life. You will feel calmer, more relaxed, and with a much clearer mind.

Give yourself a goal and a reason. Set a small challenge for yourself and win it! Set a precise number of days during which you will meditate and then find the motivation to do it. You can find the motivation by analyzing why you decided to start meditating, that is your why. For example, a good challenge might be to meditate 5 minutes a day for 21 days in the evening, if your reason for starting is to improve sleep quality or avoid insomnia. You have a very good reason to achieve your goal, and you will bring home a great victory. By the way, 5 minutes a day for 21 days is a good goal, it's a good challenge to yourself, absolutely within your reach. You might consider starting here if it doesn't seem too overwhelming. I can assure you that with a good why you can do it with no problem.

Don't judge yourself. Try to treat yourself as kindly as possible. Many people get angry and resent themselves if they make mistakes while learning to meditate. If while meditating, you find you are chasing a thought, don't get angry with yourself, just let it go and bring your attention back to the object of your meditation. You have to let go, accept whatever is happening, accept yourself, embrace yourself, and embrace the moment. Don't get nervous, just accept what comes, and be with yourself. I know it can be difficult and frustrating because you feel like you're doing it wrong or you're not really meditating, but that's okay, let go, forgive yourself, and keep trying. With time and practice, you will continue to improve and stay well focused on your meditation, you soon won't find yourself getting distracted anymore, or chasing random thoughts.

<u>Try guided meditations for initial help.</u> In this book, you will find a chapter with step-by-step transcriptions of 10 guided meditations. You will also find transcriptions of guided meditations in the chapter on "How to start meditating" and in the chapter on "Breathing and Meditation". On my YouTube channel, you will find audio versions of some of them, and as we said before, online you can find many such apps and resources. You can try them to see if they help you, at least in the beginning. If you get distracted while trying, remember the previous point, don't get upset, and keep trying. I personally, when I first started, preferred those that in an introduction explained what to do and then left background music where I could proceed in intimacy to do what was described in the introduction. In other guided meditations, the teacher guides you throughout the process. The preference for one or the other guided meditation is subjective. It is such an intimate practice that some people prefer to do the whole process alone and without guidance, which is why I left this suggestion for last. That is also why I have included step-by-step texts, to give you a

reliable and complete guide, without having to resort to guided audios, if the procedure is not for you.

The 11 Tips for Meditating Better

1. Choose the Best Time

Morning is a good time to meditate because we have just gotten up and the mind is still quite free, not clogged with all the thoughts and information that usually crowd it throughout the day. In addition, meditating in the morning allows you to carry the benefits of the practice with you throughout the day.

If you need to improve the quality of your sleep you might find it more helpful to meditate in the evening.

If, on the other hand, work stresses you out, it might be helpful to take a meditation break during the workday to find a moment to disconnect and relieve stress.

2. Choose the Best Place

It is important you meditate in a place where you feel comfortable otherwise you will find it very difficult to immerse yourself in the meditative state. It is also useful to find a quiet and peaceful place (even if you meditate in the office, I'm pretty sure you can find such a place).

When you start to become a little more experienced, to train your concentration you may want to choose a place that is not completely silent but has some noise, to train you to maintain your concentration despite this distraction.

3. Be prepared

Before you begin your practice I recommend that you drink if you are thirsty or pee if you need to. This is to prevent these circumstances from disturbing your concentration. Especially in the beginning, the fewer distractions you have, the easier it will be to get into the practice.

Clothing is also part of the preparation phase. Meditating in clothes that are comfortable and possibly made of natural fibers helps you feel more comfortable. If you meditate, for example, in the office and are wearing something constricting, loosen one or more buttons, and undo your belt or tie, so that you are relaxed and not constricted.

Don't forget your posture while getting ready. It should be comfortable and allow you to keep your back straight when you sit down. Whether on the floor or in a chair, prepare your seat with cushions appropriate for your comfort.

4. Find Your Why

Having a why when you meditate is useful for a variety of reasons. First of all, as I said in the previous chapter, it is useful because it keeps you consistent in your practice, and consistency is essential to achieve results in meditation (as in any other discipline you undertake).

Second, it is very useful for choosing your mantras, intentionalities, or what you decide to focus your meditation on. So, find your motivation, find the reason why you decided to start meditating.

5. Stop

In a fast-paced world like the one we live in, the concept of stopping may seem a bit strange and impossible. However, you need it to feel good. You also need it to meditate better.

You need to try to stop the avalanche of information that the world around you tries to send to your brain every second. Try to stop your thoughts during the day and pay attention to what you are doing. It will come in handy during meditation.

When you walk to the bus stop after work, turn off your phone, put it in your bag, and try to walk without thinking about anything in particular. While you are cleaning, put your usual gestures into motion without thinking about anything in particular. These little breaks given to your mind will help you meditate better, and you will also feel the benefit throughout the day. They are a bit like active little meditations, like when you practice yoga or run. Take a break from the hustle and bustle of the world and try to be present in the "here and now."

6. Remember that You Are a Spiritual Being

It is often the hectic pace of the world around us that makes us forget that we are spiritual beings living in a physical body. The world around us puts all the focus on our physical side and we end up forgetting the spiritual side.

To be well, you need a perfect balance between the two. If this balance is not in place, you feel incomplete, and fail to fulfill yourself.

Try to listen to both the needs of your body and your spirit, this will help you meditate better and maintain the balance in a stable way to feel good, complete, and fulfilled.

7. Focus on an Object

Training this practice in your daily life will be very helpful for you to focus better during meditation.

Choose an object that has meaning or significance to you and focus your attention on it for a few days. Using your senses explore it, but keep your attention on it only, and do it at least once a day. Focus on its color, its smell, and its texture to your touch. Does it have a taste? Does it reproduce a sound?

Use the power of focus and learn to concentrate. It will benefit you in your daily life and in meditation practice.

8. Perceive the Essence of the Object

After your focus and careful exploration of your chosen object, try to imagine its history.

Who produced it? Who touched it? Where did the materials that make it come from? Dig to find its true essence.

This search will send you deep into the nature of the object you are exploring and it will be a useful and important lesson for your meditation. During the practice, in fact, you have to go deeper and deeper inside yourself until you get in touch with your essence and with your true self. This object exercise will help you in your meditation practice.

9. Breathe

I have devoted a whole chapter to the relationship between breath and meditation, but I think in the tips for meditating better it is worth emphasizing its importance again.

Often, when you start meditating, you are plagued by various negative feelings. It may be that you start meditating to get rid of anxiety, fear, guilt, anger, sadness, or depression. These negative states, characterized by high tension, certainly do not make it easy for beginners to start. Breathing can really make a profound difference. Breathing correctly strongly helps to manage negative emotions. So, breathing slowly, calmly, and deeply will calm you down enough to get into the practice easier and to slip easier into the meditative state.

10. Don't be discouraged

If on your first attempts, you find it difficult to relax and clear your mind, and you keep getting distracted by a thought, it is because your mind is very active and thinks too much because of too many surrounding stimuli. I will elaborate on this concept in the next chapter, where I will be focusing on the most common mistakes.

It is important not to get discouraged and keep trying. With persistence and the various tips I share with you in this book, you will slowly begin to stay focused longer on the object of your meditation and you will notice when an extraneous thought is about to distract you, so you can let it flow without stopping it.

I repeat: Anyone can meditate!

11. Don't Give Yourself Deadlines

Don't give yourself deadlines by which you must have "learned" to meditate and time frames by which you expect to "see" the first results. These deadlines would end up generating a state of tension that would only complicate your approaches to meditation.

Learning to do anything well takes time and perseverance, and meditation is no exception. The problem is that the society we live in is primarily based on "everything right away" and on short-term results, so this may distort your perceptions.

Take as much time as you need and don't give yourself unnecessary deadlines.

The 13 Most Common Mistakes

In this chapter, I would like to address with you what I think are the biggest obstacles a beginner faces when deciding to start meditating. I am referring to those circumstances that make you say, "I don't know how to meditate," "It's not for me," or "I've tried, but I can't do it."

As I stated at the end of the introduction to this book: everyone can meditate and everyone should meditate. Everyone can do it; all it takes is the mind to meditate, and we all have one. Unfortunately, it is your mental schemes that hinder you in the process because they try to convince you that you are not capable. Your mental patterns keep telling you that you are making mistakes, that you are not doing it the right way, and that you should give up because you are not progressing at all. You listen to all this and you end up giving up. That's why I told you in the section on "Tips for getting started in meditation" that you should not judge yourself, so as not to trigger this mechanism.

Since I hear these negative statements too often, I decided to address the problem by defining the most common mistakes, to help you avoid falling into them or to get out of them promptly, should they happen to you. Let's see what prevents you from practicing correctly and why you are not getting all the benefits you can.

1. Your Mind is Too Restless

Just as it is true that during your day your mind is affected by the quality of your meditation, the opposite is also true. The amount of useless and stressful material you crowd your mind with every day and keep it occupied with, affects the quality of your meditation.

Meditation, I repeat, is a means to quiet your mind and keep its hectic activity in check. But, how can 5 minutes of meditation every now and then keep in check hours and hours of negative stimuli, mental stress, restlessness, and everything else you allow in into your mind for at least 12 hours a day every day? It would be like eating fast-food every day and expecting to weigh like a feather.

You should observe your mind during the day, try to understand what goes into it, and filter out some of the negative stimuli, for your own good. This will make it easier to meditate, and the better you meditate the calmer your mind will become, feeding a healthy circle that will bring you immediate benefits.

A mind that is too busy leads to the second problem.

2. Too Much Information

Most of what crowds your mind and makes it agitated and always busy comes from screens, which we have become accustomed to being glued to all day long. Social media, games, movies, news, blog articles, and I could go on much longer with this list.

In short, we expose our minds and brains to a flood of information for a very large number of hours every day, and when we sit down to meditate, our brains are in fervent activity. All this information gives us ideas, creates images and visions, and our brain and mental activity are overwhelmed with agitation.

Not only that, what is broadcasted on your screens is specifically designed to stimulate an emotional reaction in you, particularly related to 4 negative emotions: fear, anger, restlessness, and desire. Those 4 emotions agitate your mind as you try to learn how to meditate.

Again, how can a few minutes of sporadic attempts to learn how to meditate get the better out of hours of daily content that leverage such totalizing emotions?

You should analyze the emotions you feel when you consume certain content and, if you are stimulated by these negative emotions, you should reduce your viewing. This will improve your mental state and make it easier for you to deal with your first approaches to meditation, triggering the beneficial circle I mentioned earlier. You will meditate better, your mind will be calmer, and less hectic throughout the day, then you will meditate even better, and so on until you achieve inner peace and well-being in your life. You will be less stressed, more productive, and less distracted; you will be present in the "here and now."

These first two issues introduce the third.

3. You are Not Very Constant

Every day your mind is occupied with this huge amount of information and you often don't even find the constancy to meditate every day. It really only takes a few minutes a day to start getting results, but you don't find them, however, I bet you make time for your favorite social! It is time to choose and that is why I told you in the previous chapter that you need to find your why, you need a reason to be consistent.

To be permanently effective in your life, meditation must be practiced daily. If you sit and meditate once in a while you might enjoy some benefit on a physical level, but if you want real change in your life on a physical, mental, spiritual, and emotional level, you need daily constancy.

It really only takes even 2 or 3 minutes at first, but those 2 or 3 minutes have to be every single day because you have to develop a habit. This is how human beings function, we function by habits, we do what we do because we are used to doing it, and meditation has to become your habit.

Are your days too busy? Get up 5 minutes earlier! Not sure if you are doing it right? It doesn't matter, do it anyway, sooner or later you will get better. Not sure which technique you prefer? Pick one and get started. Nothing should stop your determination to meditate for 2 or 3 minutes daily.

You will see that slowly and without any effort on your part, those 2 or 3 minutes will become 5, then 10, and this too will start a positive circle of events. You will meditate better and without realizing it you will meditate longer, you will feel better, and meditate even better, and so on. So, your watchword is **CONSISTENCY**.

The fourth problem arises from a mix of the first three. Too much mental stimulation, too little constancy, and yet very high expectations.

4. You Have Unrealistic Expectations

It is right to start meditating because you are attracted by the benefits meditation brings to your life. It is wrong, however, to have unrealistic expectations and also to put all the focus on those expectations.

Until you seriously work on the first three mistakes mentioned you won't be able to see great results, so try not to fall into the mistake of giving up because you don't see the hoped-for benefits. It is just a matter of time, practice, and adjusting a few things along the way.

To solve this problem, it can help you not to put too much focus on expectations related to results. Try to focus on the pleasure that meditating gives you, and make the practice a fun, enjoyable time where you feel good.

5. You Don't Prepare Yourself

Many people struggle to enter a meditative state because they do not prepare to meditate. I have said many times that it only takes a few minutes a day to meditate, so don't expect a lot of preparation. It really only takes small gestures but they can make all the difference.

In step three of the steps on "How to start meditating", I indicated to you to take 3 deep breaths inhaling through the nose and exhaling through the mouth. This gesture is preparation because it relaxes and calms you, helps you to enter the meditative state more easily, and lets you go deeper with your meditation.

Some people prefer to state their intention instead of breathing, others need to stretch their muscles and loosen contractures, or practice various combinations of these three suggestions. You can experiment to find the best solution for you, the important thing is to prepare yourself in some way.

6. Too Much Confusion about Techniques

I devoted an entire chapter of this book to discussing the most popular meditation techniques and one chapter to recommending you a technique to start with.

Everyone is different, however, so once you have experimented with how to get started you should spend the first few weeks testing which technique is easiest for you to apply and which gives you the most results. Let's say that one week of testing each technique should be enough, and in just over a month you should have found your ideal solution.

Beginners often do not do this path of test and analysis. Therefore, they find themselves jumping from one technique to another with little benefit after months of attempts.

It is essential to find your technique and dedicate yourself to it for an appropriate amount of time. You can evaluate changes and variations when your experience begins to grow, but doing so at the beginning proves to be a mistake and a hindrance. You can't master any technique because you don't give yourself the time to do so and therefore you believe you are not capable of meditating.

Repetition of a technique, whether it is focusing on a chakra, mantra, or breath, makes you gain more intimacy and affinity with the technique itself. It will become easier and easier for you to practice it, your meditation will become deeper and deeper, and you will get better and better results.

So, give yourself a few weeks to choose the technique and then focus only on the chosen one.

7. You Doubt Too Much

As I mentioned in mistake 6, when you go from one technique to another and see no results, you start to persuade yourself that you are not capable of meditating. This doubt and self-criticism, in addition to demotivating you, tend to distract you during your practice.

Try not to judge yourself, especially during practice. As you practice, let yourself go, immerse yourself in meditation, and don't think about whether you are doing it right or wrong. Just do it.

All you have to do is focus your attention on the breath, a mantra, or a chakra and hold this attention as long as possible. When it fails, as soon as you notice it, bring it back to where you want it to be. At first, your attention will be short-lived and it will take you a while to notice that it is wandering, but with practice, you will hold it longer and longer and notice a lot quicker when it begins to wander.

No judgments, no doubts, just keep repeating this process, and your results will come. It may sound simplistic, but the gist of meditation is all here, in the brief process of keeping your attention as long as possible on the chosen object, and bringing it back as soon as you notice that something has distracted your concentration.

8. You Punish Yourself

A consequential mistake of doubting and judging yourself is that you punish yourself in some way. When a thought comes to distract you during meditation, you berate yourself.

Don't! It doesn't help your meditation and it doesn't help you. When a thought comes to distract you, welcome it, let it flow, and watch it go away without reproaching yourself for anything. Then, return your attention to the object of your meditation.

9. You Do not Practice with Attention

If you practice superficially and without paying due attention to your gestures, it is normal to find it hard to get into a meditative state, and you will hardly see any results. While practicing, you need to set aside thoughts such as the things you will have to do during the day. You have to concentrate only on meditation in that handful of minutes devoted to it; you have the rest of the day for other thoughts.

I think it's easy for you to understand this point because it applies a little bit to anything you do. If you do something carelessly and listlessly, you cannot expect results in any area.

10. You Don't Practice with Intention

You must practice meditation not only with attention but also with the intention to make it deeper and deeper. If you lack this element, you will find it difficult to find the necessary calm and commit yourself to the practice daily.

Try not to experience meditation as one of the many tasks of the day. Practice it with the intention of making an important gesture for you, the most important gesture of your day. It is an appointment with yourself and your well-being. Living it with this intentionality and with this kind of reverence will help you become better and better at it.

11. You Have no Patience

Certainly, meditation will help you develop this virtue, but you have to be patient if you want to learn to meditate.

You have to be patient with yourself and with the practice. You can and will get incredible results, but it will take time.

12. You Confuse Meditation and Relaxation

To meditate you have to relax, but, as I explained in the chapter on what meditation is, you have to "achieve a state of peace while still remaining alert." This means that meditating and relaxing are not synonymous.

To meditate properly you have to create a state of balance between relaxing and being alert. Do not confuse the two terms, otherwise by using relaxation as the only parameter, you might think you are not meditating, when in fact you are.

13. You Have Negative Thoughts

Many people think they are not meditating because some negative thought happens to cross their mind. Meditation helps you deal with negativity, and over time you will see the results. However, especially in the beginning, it is normal for some negative thoughts to cross your mind.

Don't worry about it and don't dwell on it. Just let it flow as you do with all other thoughts and stay focused on the object of your meditation. If you find that you dwell on it, don't reproach yourself, don't judge yourself, move on, let it go, and bring your attention back to the object of your meditation.

Step-By-Step Meditations

At this point in the book, you have enough information to successfully take your first steps into the world of meditation, and also a good amount of suggestions for moving to a more advanced level.

In this chapter, I would like to address meditation suggestions based on the time you have available or the purpose for which you are meditating. I will divide each practice into numbered steps and give you the outline of various guided meditations to make your approaches to the practice even easier.

On my YouTube channel, whose link is in the introduction, I often post guided meditations that you can follow, but having this written option has two additional functions. As I mentioned to you earlier, guided meditations are useful for beginners, especially those who are just starting out. However, this is not a truth that applies to everyone. For some, meditation is a very intimate process and, especially in the beginning, you want to do it in absolute solitude. For me, for example, this was the case. My first few times were in absolute solitude and autonomy, with time and experience, I was able to open myself to the teachings of a master and his guided meditations.

The second strength of these transcriptions is that they allow you to maintain intimacy while still giving you the precise directions you need, and you can leverage this information in two ways.

You can memorize the various passages and then perform them later. Or, with the voice recorder on your cell phone, you can record yourself slowly reading the various steps and build your own guided meditation, with your own voice and your own meditation times. As your only caution, I recommend that you allow time between steps to apply what you describe. In this way, you will also create a meditation of a length equivalent to the time you set for your practice, whereas in classic guided ones, the time is not set by you and, especially in the beginning, they can be a bit too long and tiring.

Well, if you are ready, let's begin.

Short Meditation - 1 Minute

Let's start with a very short meditation. It is simple and you can easily practice it every day. It only takes 1 minute to practice it and you do it by creating a connection with yourself and your breath. With regular practice, you will soon see the first benefits in your life.

You can also practice it for more than 1 minute, of course. However, even one minute repeated every single day will give you a deep sense of calm and balance and help you center and ground yourself.

Here are the steps to follow:

1. Sit on the floor, with your legs crossed and your back straight (with all your Chakras aligned), but relaxed. (If you prefer to sit on a chair or use a cushion that's okay too, just follow the directions in the chapter on "How to start meditating"). You need to be comfortable, but not too comfortable because you need to remain alert.

2. Shoulders relaxed, chest open, and hands laying on your thighs or knees.

3. Close your eyes. Breathe through your nose.

4. Focus on your breathing.

5. Start breathing in a controlled way and count the duration of your breath. Breathe in one, slow, deep stream, and make inhalation and exhalation the same time length. I recommend 3 or 4 seconds (for me 4

seconds is perfect). So, for example, inhale for 4 seconds and exhale for 4 seconds, then again. Inhale for 4 seconds and then exhale for 4 seconds. Continue ...

6. Focus all your attention on this count and let the breathing absorb you completely. Continue for one minute or as long as you decided to devote yourself to meditation. You are now breathing in a well-balanced way. As you follow the flow of your breath, feel the air entering your nose and reaching your whole body, and then leaving it as you exhale. Following your breath brings you into the present moment, into the "here and now", and infuses your body and spirit with calm and peace, making you feel grounded and balanced. Following your breath brings you into the present moment, centers, and roots you, and as you proceed with the practice, you feel it more and more deeply. Feel the balance between your body and mind.

7. Start by slowly moving the fingers of your hands to gradually move out of the state and go back to your body. Then slowly open your eyes. Before getting up, take a second to enjoy the feelings of peace, tranquility, and balance that you have generated, so that they will follow you as long as possible throughout your day, making it a better day.

The incredible advantage of this short meditation is that you can practice it virtually anywhere. In the office, sitting at your desk. On the subway, sitting on your way to work. At home, returning from a hard day. During a break, during an anxious moment, or during a particularly nerve-wracking or stressful circumstance. Allowing yourself to be completely absorbed by the breath as this meditation teaches you to do will calm you down, and give you the balance you need to deeply enjoy your day.

Short Meditation - 3 Minutes

This is another practice that aims to bring peace, serenity, and balance to your body and mind quickly. It only takes 3 minutes a day, every day, but, again, you can practice for as long as you want.

Here are the steps to follow:

1. Sit on the floor with your legs crossed and your back straight (with all your Chakras aligned), but not stiff. Relax your shoulders. (If you prefer to sit on a chair or use a cushion that's okay too, just follow the directions in the chapter on "How to start meditating"). You need to be comfortable, but not too comfortable because you need to remain alert.

2. Close your eyes. Breathe through your nose.

3. Shoulders relaxed, chest open, and hands laying on your thighs or knees.

4. Do not control your breathing. Breathe normally, and let your breath flow naturally.

5. Watch your breath flow because it brings you into the present moment, into the "here and now." Through the breath, relax your body, and let go of all tension. Do not hold any tension, let it go with your breath.

6. Keep observing your breath going in and out of your body. Visualize the exact process of the air entering your nose and traveling throughout your body when you inhale, and then leaving when you exhale. Continue for 3 minutes to stay focused on this observation and visualization of the air going in and out of your body.

7. If during this observation of your breath you get distracted or any thoughts come into your mind, that's okay. As soon as you notice it, bring your attention back to your breath and to your visualization of the air coming in through your nose, going through your whole body, and then leaving your body through your nostrils.

8. Start slowly moving your fingers on your hands to gradually come out of the state and return to your body.

Then slowly open your eyes. Before getting up, take a second to enjoy the feelings of peace, tranquility, and balance that you have generated, so that they will follow you as long as possible throughout your day, making it a better day.

Short Meditation - 5 Minutes

This practice too aims to bring peace, serenity, and balance to body and mind, pretty quickly. It only takes 5 minutes a day, every day, but, again, you can practice for as long as you want.

Here are the steps to follow:

1. Sit on the floor with your legs crossed and your back straight (with all your Chakras aligned), but not stiff. Relax your shoulders. (If you prefer to sit on a chair or use a cushion that's okay too, just follow the directions in the chapter on "How to start meditating"). You need to be comfortable, but not too comfortable because you need to remain.

2. Close your eyes. Breathe through your nose.

3. Shoulders relaxed, chest open, and hands laying on your thighs or knees.

4. Do not control your breathing. Breathe normally, and let your breath flow naturally.

5. Watch your breath flow because it brings you into the present moment, into the "here and now", and brings you awareness.

6. As you observe your breath flow, you can feel the air around you protecting you, wrapping around you, and supporting you.

7. As you watch your breath flow, you can feel the connection with Mother Earth supporting and protecting you. You can feel Her under you if you are sitting on the ground or under your feet if you are in a chair.

8. As you watch your breath flow, feel protected and supported by the Air and the Earth. Stay focused and concentrated on these sensations throughout your practice.

9. Begin by slowly moving the fingers of your hands to gradually move out of the state and back to your body. Then slowly open your eyes. Before getting up, take a second to enjoy the feelings of peace, tranquility, and balance that you have generated, so that they will follow

you as long as possible throughout your day and make it a better day.

All three of these practices can be practiced for different lengths of time. The real difference lies in which of the three makes you feel more comfortable and allows you to enter a meditative state more easily: breath control, observing your breath, or focusing on sensations. Testing the various methods will help you get to know yourself better and clearly understand what works for you.

Short Meditation for Gratitude - 5 Minutes

It only takes 5 minutes a day, every day, but, again, you can practice it for as long as you want. It is very similar to the other meditations already described, with the difference that you give yourself an intention, we might say a purpose. For example, your intention might be to be present, to be the observer of your breath, to be the observer of your energy, the observer of your body sensations, and so on. This practice brings calm, inner peace, and deep gratitude.

Here are the steps to follow:

1. Sit on the floor with your legs crossed and your back straight (with all your Chakras aligned), but not stiff. Relax your shoulders. (If you prefer to sit on a chair or use a cushion that's okay too, just follow the directions in

the chapter on "How to start meditating"). You need to be comfortable, but not too comfortable because you need to remain alert.

2. Close your eyes. Breathe through your nose.

3. Shoulders relaxed, face relaxed, chest open, and hands laying on thighs or knees.

4. Do not control your breathing. Breathe normally and let the breath flow naturally.

5. Watch your breath flow because it brings you into the present moment, into the "here and now", and makes you feel centered and grounded.

6. Bring your hands together in front of your chest and state your intention for this meditation. It could be, for example, to be present in the "here and now," present to yourself and your spirit. Choose your intention.

7. Become an observer of the present moment without judging yourself and state your intention, around or on your mind (whichever makes you more comfortable). Now you can put your hands back on your thighs or knees.

8. Go back to observing your breath, observing each time the air goes in and out of your body. Leave it natural and relaxed, just observe it. If you get distracted or a thought comes to your mind, bring your attention back to observing your breath as soon as you notice your distraction. Do this with intention, without judging, or punishing yourself.

9. Continue to observe your breath, bring your attention back to it throughout the practice, and allow the practice to make you feel peaceful and calm.

10. Before concluding the practice, bring your joined hands back to your heart level and express gratitude for all the reasons for gratitude that certainly abound in your life and that you can surely see more clearly in this state. Then carry all this gratitude with you after the practice and throughout your day.

11. Take a deep breath. Smile. Begin to slowly move your fingers to gradually come out of the state and return to your body. Then slowly open your eyes. Before getting up, take a second to enjoy the feelings of peace, calm, and gratitude that you have generated, so that they will follow you as long as possible throughout your day, making it a better day.

Short Morning Meditation - 3 Minutes

To start your day in the best way possible.

Here are the steps to follow:

1. Sit on the floor with your legs crossed and your back straight (with all your Chakras aligned), but not stiff. Relax your shoulders. (If you prefer to sit on a chair or use a cushion that's okay too, just follow the directions in the chapter on "how to start meditating"). You need to be comfortable, but not too comfortable because you need to remain alert.

2. Close your eyes. Breathe through your nose.

3. Shoulders relaxed, face relaxed, chest open, and hands laying on thighs or knees.

4. Do not control your breathing. Breathe normally and let your breath flow naturally.

5. Watch your breath flow through your body. Observe the air entering and leaving your body. Observe how cool the one entering your nose is and how warm the one coming out is. Observe the whole journey that oxygen makes through your body and takes root in it. Bring all your

attention inward, to the breath. This will root you in the present moment, into the "here and now".

6. Now observe the sensations generated in your body. Analyze each part of your body and how it feels to be in contact with the Earth underneath you, or the air around you. What sensations do those parts feel? They should all be pleasant sensations. If you feel a tightening somewhere, you need to control your breath and send your breath where you feel that knot. Your breath can loosen the knot and create a relaxed space in its place.

7. Feel present in your body, in your spirit, and into the world. Find yourself. Be present and aware. Practice this meditation for at least 3 minutes or as long as you like.

8. Take a deep breath. Smile. Start slowly moving your fingers on your hands to gradually come out of the state and return to your body. Then slowly open your eyes. Before getting up, take a second to enjoy the relaxing sensations you have generated, keep smiling, and let the smile and the relaxation follow you to get your day off to the best possible start.

Meditation for Better Sleep - Short - 5 Minutes

This short meditation prepares you for sleep and helps you enjoy deep sleep because it empties the mind and relaxes the body. It should be practiced just before going to sleep. It is very useful for those who struggle to get to sleep, those who have little restful sleep, those who cannot leave behind the weight of the day, and those whose minds are very active even when it is time to go to bed. It only takes 5 minutes of daily practice to improve the quality of your sleep but you can practice it even longer, depending on your needs. I recommend not practicing it by already lying down in bed. You should always practice it in a sitting position so that your chakras are aligned and your energy can flow freely.

Here are the steps to follow:

1. Sit on the floor with your legs crossed and your back straight (with all your Chakras aligned), but not stiff. Relax your shoulders. (If you prefer to sit on a chair or use a pillow that's okay too, just follow the directions in the chapter on "How to start meditating"). You need to be comfortable.

2. Close your eyes. Breathe through your nose.

3. Shoulders relaxed, face relaxed, chest open, and hands laying on your thighs or knees.

4. Do not control your breathing. Breathe normally and let your breath flow naturally.

5. Feel your body relax with your breath. Each time you exhale feel your body relax and your shoulders lower toward the ground.

6. Then, each time you exhale, bring softness into your body. Feel your joints become softer, all the tissues of your body, and then all your muscles from top to bottom. Feel your face soften when you exhale, feel your shoulders soften when you exhale, and also the heart area. Continuing down, feel your abdomen soften when you exhale, then your legs, and your feet.

7. Keep breathing flowing naturally, feel this sensation of softness throughout your body, and every time you exhale let go of any residual tension and throw all your tensions out of your body. Let go of the events of the day, especially the ones you didn't enjoy. Let go of the list of things you couldn't complete that are waiting for you tomorrow. Stop thinking about the things you didn't do as you would have liked, let them go too.

8. When you have let go of everything, welcome gratitude for all that your body has allowed you to do, and experience this deep sense of gratitude. Connect to this gratitude, feel love toward it, and toward yourself. Be grateful and in love with yourself, your mind, your body, and your soul. Continue to feel this deep gratitude until the end of the practice by going deeper and deeper into yourself as your breathing continues to flow naturally. Every time you exhale you throw out all the tensions and everything you no longer need.

9. When you feel ready, slowly open your eyes, rise slowly, and try to maintain the state you are in. Go immediately to bed. As you walk towards it keep feeling gratitude, love, and peace. When you are in bed, go back to visualizing your breath, visualize yourself throwing out everything you don't need or want, and continue until you fall asleep.

Meditation to Reduce Anxiety - Short - 5 Minutes

The purpose of this meditation is to abandon fear and feel safe. Fear and feeling unsafe are the two main conditions that trigger anxiety. In this meditation, you will let go of those two negative feelings and regain mental calm. You only need a consistent practice of 5 minutes a day to improve your anxious state and the level of stress in your life. You will also find it very useful to practice it before a situation that usually makes you anxious, for example, an interview with the boss, a date with a new potential partner, a sport or social event where you need to perform at your best, or even an exam.

Here are the steps to follow:

1. Sit on the floor with your legs crossed and your back straight (with all your Chakras aligned), but not stiff. Relax your shoulders. (If you prefer to sit on a chair or use a cushion that's okay too, just follow the directions in the chapter on "How to start meditating"). You need to be comfortable, but not too comfortable because you need to remain alert.

2. Close your eyes. Breathe through your nose.

3. Shoulders relaxed, face relaxed, chest open, and hands laying on thighs or knees.

4. Do not control your breathing. Breathe normally and let your breath flow naturally.

5. Watch your breath flow because it brings you into the present moment, into the "here and now", and makes you feel centered and grounded. Focus on your breath and

feel the muscles in your body relax with your breath. Breathe in and, when you exhale, throw out all the tension. Become soft and begin to distinctly sense the floor beneath you and the air brushing against your skin, and surrounding your body.

6. Now that you perceive the boundaries of your body, begin to visualize a blue light coming closer and closer to you until it embraces you completely. Now, the boundaries of your body are completely wrapped in this blue light. The blue light is a safe place, a place where you are not afraid. Stay here, wrapped in the safe blue light for as long as you need. If a thought comes to distract you, let it go, and come back here, to your safe place. Stay focused on the blue light that surrounds you and feel the peace, calm, and safety it gives you for as long as you feel you need it.

7. Begin to slowly move the fingers of your hands to gradually come out of the state and then return to your body. Then slowly open your eyes. Before getting up, take a second to enjoy the feelings of peace, calm, and security that you have generated, so that they will follow you as long as possible throughout your day, making it a better day.

Meditation to Reduce Stress - 10 Minutes

The deep connection that this meditation creates causes you to feel centered, and grounded, and calms your mind. In such a state, you start to feel free from the grip of stress and will easily manage violent emotions such as anger or nervousness. Those bad emotions are often characterized by rigid body posture and negative thoughts crowding your mind like you couldn't push them away. The relaxation of body and mind that are given by this meditation allows you to better manage these negative aspects, push away negative thoughts easily, and bring positive benefits into your life throughout your day. With daily repetition, you will reduce stress in your life and live a happier life. This technique is very useful for learning to let go of everything you need to let go of.

Here are the steps to follow:

1. Sit on the floor with your legs crossed and your back straight (with all your Chakras aligned), but not stiff. Relax your shoulders. (If you prefer to sit on a chair or use a cushion that's okay too, just follow the directions in the chapter on "How to start meditating"). You need to be comfortable, but not too comfortable because you need to remain alert.

2. Close your eyes. Breathe through your nose.

3. Shoulders relaxed, face relaxed, chest open, and hands laying on your thighs or knees.

4. Start focusing on yourself the moment you close your eyes. Let go of other thoughts. Let go of distractions.

5. Concentrate and focus on your breath so that the mind starts to calm down. Follow your breath and focus on yourself until you feel connected to your deepest inner part.

6. Bring all your attention to your body. Observe your back. It is straight, with the Chakras aligned, but not rigid. Your face, shoulders, and arms are relaxed. Observe your chest as it opens and expands with each inhalation.

7. Bring your attention back to your breath and observe its flow. Do not try to control it, let it flow spontaneously, and naturally. Observe the air entering your nose when you inhale and leaving when you exhale. Exhale gently. Visualize your breath making its journey through your body.

8. Each time you exhale, let go of all that is negative, all that no longer serves you, and all that you need to let go of. Keep your attention on observing your breath throughout your meditation and feel yourself letting go each time you

exhale. If a thought or something else comes to distract your attention, don't worry, and don't judge yourself. Just let go of the distraction, watch it as it passes, as it proceeds to go past, and bring your attention back to the breath observation.

9. While you observe your breath, you will begin to feel present and connected in the "here and now" because you will begin to sense the boundaries of your body, the earth where it rests, and the air that surrounds and embraces it.

10. Start by slowly moving the fingers of your hands to gradually move out of the state and then back to the body. Then slowly open your eyes. Before getting up, take a second to enjoy the sensations you have generated. Try to feel what has changed in you after this meditation. Take in all the sensations and emotions that come in both body and mind and bring them with you throughout your day.

TIP: This meditation is very useful for stimulating the Third Eye Chakra. To do this, you will only need to slightly modify the phase of coming out of this meditative state. At step 10, after starting to move your fingers, rub your hands together until your palms are warm. Then bring your hands together, joined as if in prayer, and raise them to forehead height. Place your thumbs in the space between the eyebrows and begin massaging the area with small concentric movements. Continue for a minute or two, then slowly open your eyes and proceed with the rest of the directions in step ten. This gesture will lengthen your meditation by a few minutes but will bring additional benefits to your life and well-being.

Mind-Body Connection Meditation - 5 Minutes

This practice helps you to connect your body and mind. It gives you a strong awareness of yourself, your body, your spiritual energy, and your immense and infinite potential. It is very useful for those who have problems with insecurity, fragility, and vulnerability because it helps the connection with the true and perfect self and its infinite energy. It is also very useful for balancing and energizing your Chakras, as the visualization you practice runs through your body's energy centers activating and stimulating them.

Here are the steps to follow:

1. Sit on the floor with your legs crossed and your back straight (with all your Chakras aligned), but not stiff. Relax your shoulders. (If you prefer to sit on a chair or use a cushion that's okay too, just follow the directions in the chapter on "How to start meditating"). You need to

be comfortable, but not too comfortable because you need to remain alert.

2. Close your eyes. Breathe through your nose.

3. Shoulders relaxed, face relaxed, chest open, and hands laying on thighs or knees. Arms are also relaxed so don't keep them stiff.

4. Bring attention to your breath and observe its flow. Don't try to control it, let it flow spontaneously, and naturally. Observe the air entering your nose when you inhale and leaving when you exhale. Breathe in a gentle, light, calm, and relaxed way. Visualize the breath making its journey through your body.

5. As you continue to observe the breath, begin to look inside yourself. Bring all your attention to the space in the center of your head. Slowly descend through your body keeping your attention on this journey. Bring your attention to your throat, then your chest, your heart, continue down to reach your navel, then your pelvis, and finally the part in contact with the ground. Keep constant awareness of this path, and when you have reached your bottom, slowly begin to walk back this same path the other way around, from your bottom to the top of your head.

6. When you have returned to the center of your head become aware that you are in a special place, through which you express your true being and your uniqueness. Gain a deeper and deeper awareness of your body and perceive it as it expands into the surrounding reality. Feel your immense greatness and your energy spreading everywhere.

7. Now your physical body is totally relaxed and deeply connected to your internal energy, and to your mind.

8. Begin to slowly move the fingers of your hands to gradually come out of the state and return to your body. Then slowly open your eyes. Before getting up, take a second to enjoy the sensations you have generated so that they will follow you as long as possible throughout your day, making it a better day.

Meditation to Calm Your Mind - 10 Minutes

Calming your mind is essential for maintaining well-being in times of stress, anxiety, or when you are affected by a negative or emotionally frustrating event. This practice is therefore very useful in a varied number of circumstances, for example, for those who work in a difficult and competitive environment, for those who are experiencing a difficult relationship, for those who are having difficulties in their relationships with their family, and in general, in all those situations that generate negative feelings that cause anxiety, stress, outbursts of anger, or feelings of unmotivated sadness. The practice involves the recitation of the "Sacred Mantra of Breath". The empty space between the recitation of the two verses of the mantra creates a deep sense of peace, which is why this technique succeeds in calming the mind so effectively.

Here are the steps to follow:

1. Sit on the floor with your legs crossed and your back straight (with all your Chakras aligned), but not stiff. Relax your shoulders. (If you prefer to sit on a chair or use a cushion that's okay too, just follow the directions in the chapter on "How to start meditating"). You need to be comfortable, but not too comfortable because you need to remain alert.

2. Close your eyes. Breathe through your nose.

3. Shoulders relaxed, face relaxed, chest open, and hands laying on thighs or knees. Arms are also relaxed so don't keep them stiff.

4. Relax your whole body, trying to ground, and center yourself in this relaxed position.

5. Bring your attention to your breath and observe its flow. Don't try to control it, let it flow spontaneously, and naturally. Observe the air entering your nose when you inhale and leaving when you exhale. Breathe in a gentle, light, calm, and relaxed way. Visualize the breath making its journey through your body.

6. As your breath flows freely, begin to visualize a beach at the sea or lake. Observe the water and its fluidity. Be inspired by this element, by its fluidity, by the way, it always adapts to circumstances, and also by its strength and energy. Visualize the water enveloping you. This element is outside and inside you.

7. Keep observing your breath and associate a mantra with it. The sacred mantra of breath is "I AM". When you inhale, mentally pronounce "I", and when you exhale, mentally pronounce "AM". Mentally repeat the mantra with each breath. (TIP: For the beneficial effects of the mantra to occur you must keep a constant focus on your breath and bring back your attention immediately in case of any distraction. In addition, you can also use the original Sanskrit version of the mantra, which is "SO HAM", meaning precisely "I AM THIS". You will mentally repeat "SO" when you inhale and "HAM" when you exhale).

8. The mantra enters the body, goes through it, and flows through it. It is like a wave of water flowing through you with all its energy. Proceed with mental repetition of the mantra throughout the practice. Keep hearing it and visualizing it as a wave flowing through you, while keeping your attention on your breath. The sound of the mantra repeated in your mind sounds like a whisper produced by a little wave. This sound brings you to the present moment and you become the mantra.

9. Before leaving the state, let go of the mantra slowly and stay in your breath for a few seconds (count at least three deep breaths).

10. Start moving the fingers of your hands slowly to gradually exit the meditation state and return to your body. Then open your eyes slowly. Before getting up, take a second to enjoy the feelings you have generated so that they will follow you as long as possible throughout your day, making it a better day. Feel gratitude for yourself because you have taken time to devote to yourself, your well-being, and inner peace, bringing enormous benefit to your life.

TIP: You may find it pleasing to put audio in the background that reproduces the sound of waves of a calm sea.

Conclusion

Here we are at the end of this journey together!

I would really like to thank you for following me this far, and I hope it has been as enjoyable for you to go through this journey together as it has been for me to lead you to the discovery of the wonderful world of meditation and your inner power.

You now possess all the knowledge to begin practicing meditation successfully and unlock your inner power. I hope you have already started to test and look for the practice that suits you better.

Do not treat this book as pure entertainment or a means to satisfy a curiosity, please use it as the tool it is intended to be. I have written it to enable you to bring all the incredible benefits of meditation into your life in an easy way, and I really hope you will.

I would love to hear what you think of this book and if it has helped you in any way. A review would certainly be appreciated, but you can also contact me directly by email: comesbloccareituoichakra@gmail.com

You can also reach me on my YouTube channel, where you can write me in the comments of any video:

https://www.youtube.com/channel/UC5DxslTyhtdH5iQo1UtkO9Q

My channels are mainly in Italian because I am Italian and I started my teachings in my own country. Anyhow, feel free to write me in English. In fact, I am in touch with loads of English-speaking people that bought my books who seek advice now and again or enquire about new books coming out.

Finally, if you are interested in learning more about my content I leave you the link to my previous book, which I have often mentioned in various chapters. The title is, "Chakras for Beginners - A Complete Guide to Balance Your Chakras and Healing Yourself with Yoga, Meditation, Crystals, Essential Oils, and Other Self-Healing Techniques". Most of the topics are closely related to the ones I explained in this book. All my content is focused on taking care of yourself to improve the quality of your life emotionally, mentally, spiritually, and physically.

Ebook:

https://www.amazon.com/dp/B0B5PB7DB9

Paperback (color):

https://www.barnesandnoble.com/w/chakras-for-beginners-mind-body-masterclass/1141405006?ean=9781739665210

Hardcover (color):

https://www.amazon.com/dp/B0B5KV646F

Well, now it is really the time of farewells. I hope to see you again somewhere, be it an email, another book, or a video.

I wish you all the best in life,

NAMASTÉ

Anja D.

www.ingramcontent.com/pod-product-compliance
Lightning Source LLC
Chambersburg PA
CBHW050245120526
44590CB00016B/2219